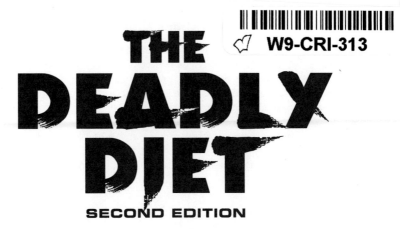

W9-CRI-313

THE DEADLY DIET

SECOND EDITION

RECOVERING FROM ANOREXIA & BULIMIA

TERENCE J. SANDBEK, PH.D.

NEW HARBINGER PUBLICATIONS, INC.

Publisher's Note

This publication is designed to provide accurate and authoritative information in regard to the subject matter covered. It is sold with the understanding that the publisher is not engaged in rendering psychological, financial, legal, or other professional services. If expert assistance or counseling is needed, the services of a competent professional should be sought.

Anyone suffering from anorexia or bulimia, or any other serious eating disorder, should use this book only under competent medical supervision. You should not attempt to treat yourself. Proper medical attention is important.

Edited by Kirk Johnson and Mary McCormick
Cover design by SHELBY DESIGNS & ILLUSTRATES

Library of Congress Catalog Card Number: 92-050707

ISBN 1-879237-43-3 Paperback
ISBN 1-879237-43-1 Hardcover

First printing 1993, 5,000

To Tim, who gave me the courage to pursue this innovative treatment program and to Andrea, who first told me about the Voice.

I would like to thank Mary McCormick for her editorial assistance.

Content

Introduction

*This book is for people who believe that being thin is the
same as being happy.*

It was 102 degrees outside in the middle of July. Roger came into my
office wearing a long-sleeved wool shirt and a sweater. He showed no
signs of the heat discomfort that the rest of the city was experiencing.
His body was so malnourished from anorexia that his metabolism had
slowed down to protect his body's loss of heat. On this sweltering day,
he was cold.

Roger, my first "real" Deadly Dieter client, had heard me lecture
about a new approach to eating disorders. After the lecture, he had asked
to see me in therapy. Since the ideas I had discussed were fairly new
(there had only been a few articles on eating disorders from a cognitive-
behavioral approach in the professional literature), I was somewhat reluctant to see him professionally. However, Roger was desperate and persistent. He had been to several large clinics at various places in the United

States. At other times, he had lapsed into a coma and had to be rushed to emergency rooms. He had just had his thirtieth birthday and saw no end in sight for the miserable life he led. He wanted to try my approach to the problem, even though it was an experimental one.

Slowly we explored our way through the myths and misunderstandings that had grown up around his Deadly Diet. We looked at his problem from the point of view that anorexia was due to a distorted perception of reality. As expected, we found that he had numerous mental misconceptions of what life was like. After only eight visits, Roger told me that he felt strong enough to terminate therapy and try it on his own. I had serious misgivings about going along with this plan because I had been told by other professionals that anorexia was one of the most tenacious mental health problems.

But since there had been significant improvement in his health, behavior, and attitude, and even some weight gain, I had no reason to keep him in therapy. We agreed that the door would be open should he need to come back. This was in 1979. I have had intermittent contact with Roger since that time. At times, it has been difficult for him to keep from slipping back into his old ways of coping with life. Nevertheless, he has successfully maintained the thirty pounds he regained. As an extremely talented artisan, he has been quite successful in his trade. During the first year I spent writing this book, he also got married.

Unfortunately, not all clients have been as quickly successful as Roger. But he gave me the courage to pursue a new cognitive-behavioral approach to the treatment of the Deadly Diet. His success soon became known to other people with the same problem, and they came to duplicate his success. Some of them made it, some of them failed. Working with them, I was able to develop and refine these techniques into a successful program for working with the Deadly Diet.

Although the mental health field has been concerned with people who have eating problems, it has generally focused attention on people who are overweight. More recently, mental health professionals have begun looking at the disorders of anorexia nervosa and bulimia. It is now difficult to pick up a popular magazine and not find an article about eating disorders. Books are being written on the topic, and there is even a professional journal dedicated entirely to studying eating disorders.

The death of Karen Carpenter in 1982 seemed to make these problems a national concern. The books and articles that followed have served a valuable purpose in educating the public about the seriousness and incidence of Deadly Diets. This information has been reassuring to thousands of people because the authors have shown that the problem is not an isolated one and have convincingly proven that people with this problem are not "sick" or "crazy," but rather normal people with a serious problem.

Unfortunately, almost all of these books and articles have been *descriptive* in nature. They have described the problem and have often done it very well. But when a person with a Deadly Diet has finished reading this information, she often wonders what to do next. Many of my clients have told me, "I was so excited when I found that article because the person in the article was just like me. I enjoyed reading about her conquering the problem. But when I got to the end of the article, I didn't know any more about how to help myself than when I started reading."

The purpose of this book will be *prescriptive* rather than descriptive. A fairly small amount of material is devoted to what the problem is and how bad it can be. Instead, this book attempts to offer proven tools and techniques that can help an individual overcome this problem. If you would like to know more about the hows and whys of eating disorders, you can check the bibliography at the end of this book.

If you are reading this book in order to help yourself overcome an eating disorder, you will quickly discover that this approach is different from other ways of dealing with anorexia and bulimia. This method has no concern for *why* you have an eating disorder (what happened to you when you were a child), or how you feel about your problem.

This book is concerned with teaching you *how* to learn the necessary skills needed to overcome the problem. If you still want to know why you have an eating problem, you can still satisfy your curiosity AFTER you have successfully overcome the problem.

The skills you will be learning in this book are fairly easy to understand, but incredibly difficult to learn and master. You will find yourself resisting learning these skills, tempted to put them off for another time. This book cannot guarantee you success; it can only guarantee you an unbelievable amount of hard work. Every individual who has come through our program has remarked at the end that it was the most difficult thing he or she had ever done. Learning these skills and overcoming these problems is not something you can do half-heartedly. You must decide to make a full-time commitment and to put your whole life, your whole soul into learning, practicing, and mastering these skills. If this program of self-change does not take a prominent place in your life, it simply will not work.

The book is designed so that you can complete a chapter in about a week (assuming that you work on the material every day). Please don't get discouraged if it takes longer. We are all different, and the important thing is that you practice your new skills every day, seven days a week, fifty-two weeks a year! Many times throughout the course of this book you will say to yourself or someone else, "But it's so hard! I'm getting so discouraged." As I remind my own clients who tell me this nearly every week, "I never said it would be easy."

Cognitive-Behavioral Therapy

A revolution is sweeping the field of mental health. For too many years, mental health professionals have been forced to act as helpers to the general population by *talking* about the past (finding out the "why") or the present (telling a person "what" to do). These two approaches have been responsible for our poor track record.

Unfortunately, some professionals in the field have not been concerned about this sad state of affairs at all. They have assumed that if a person was not helped in therapy, then he or she must be either hiding something or in some way enjoying the pain and suffering. This attitude exempts the therapist from any major responsibility in helping to solve an individual's problem. It is amazing that the public has tolerated this arrogance for as long as it has. We certainly don't expect other professionals to act this way. If I take my car to a mechanic or if I visit a dentist, I don't expect that person to ask me how I feel about the problem. I expect competent and sound advice on what to do. Generally this takes the form of what the *professional* is going to do, not what I am going to do. Of course, once the problem is taken care of, it is my responsibility to engage in preventative behavior to keep my car or teeth in as good condition as I can.

As psychologists, we must also be held accountable for what we do. We must become more active—instead of offering a lot of "uh-huhs" and paraphrases of what the client said. Why shouldn't we answer direct questions with reasonable answers? It is intolerable for a therapist to answer a question by ruling that it is untherapeutic for a client to ask a straightforward question or by responding with no more than "How do you feel about that?"

One of the major forms of therapy today is one called cognitive behavioral. The concept behind it is simple: we are what we think. Mankind has intuitively known this for most of recorded history. We have been telling each other to change our attitudes for a very long time, knowing that if a person were to do so, positive changes would follow. The cognitive-behavioral therapist also knows that if he or she can teach a client *how* to change his or her thoughts a major portion of the battle has been won.

Other scientific fields are also beginning to acknowledge the power of inner thoughts over our lives. A physician in the September 1984 issue of *Science* wrote the following words about pain and its relationship to our thinking processes:

> Pain consists of more than an intense sensory input. There must also be an interpretation of the sensation as painful. In patients with paraplegia, strong stimulation below the level of the lesion will cause reflex withdrawal of the artificial limb.

The subject may, however, be unaware that the stimulus is even present. It is difficult to consider this painful.

The perception of pain also requires a context. Memory and anticipation can affect the way a sensation is interpreted. A ballet dancer may not experience discomfort even though a bone is broken. A mild ache may be magnified greatly by a cancer patient who fears it means a recurrence.

The cerebral cortex is the major site where this type of analysis takes place. Without the cerebral cortex, complex behavioral responses may occur, including orientation to an intense stimulus, but there is no suffering; we feel there is therefore no perception of pain.

This book devotes about 80 percent of its instruction to cognitive-behavioral tools. Although the next generation may look upon these ideas as somewhat primitive, these techniques are the best we have available at the present time.

Obstacles

Denial is the biggest obstacle to overcoming an eating disorder. One of the key signs indicating that your denial level may be dangerously high is the phrase, "I can quit this anytime I want." A variation of this is, "I will change when I am ready." Sometimes just admitting that the problem exists is the most difficult part of getting better.

Although the tools and techniques you will learn in this book have been tested successfully on hundreds of individuals with severe Deadly Diets, they contain no magic or easy solutions. You will probably learn very little that is new and may even be disappointed that most of it seems like good old common sense. The difference is that this approach teaches you to *systematically* attack your eating problem in a way that is both effective and satisfying. The good news: this method is very easy to understand. But the work will be hard in the sense that you will need to set priorities on your time and activities so that EACH DAY you set aside space to complete the homework assignments.

Since the first edition of this book I have received hundreds of letters and spent additional thousands of hours working with clients who have the Deadly Diet. I have found that to be successful, you need to spend at least one hour a day using these techniques. If you don't think you have an extra hour a day, you will be surprised how easy it is to find the time. Forget about using these tools as if they were a homework assignment due the next day. Spending a solid hour's block of time at the end of the day will not do you much good. However, if you spread the hour out during the day, the benefits will be enormous. Even in an extremely busy day, you still go to the bathroom. Spending a few extra minutes will help you grab more time for yourself. Five minutes here and ten minutes there can easily give you your minimum dose.

Two words of caution. First, if you just can't get an hour in on a particular day, don't fret. As long as you can get at least an hour most days, you will do okay. Second, if you really want to speed up your progress, take more than an hour a day to learn these tools. Just as in learning any skill, there are three things to remember: practice, practice, practice.

Nothing worth having in life is very easy to get. You may be a dancer, an artist, a musician, or an athlete. I'm sure you don't expect to do well in these disciplines without a lot of hard work. The same goes for conquering your Deadly Diet. How well you do will depend on how much time you spend practicing your skills—and *not* on how long you have had the problem or how severe or how unusual the problem is. The only factor in your success or failure is how much time you give to helping yourself.

You don't even have to believe in this approach, because it is based on scientific principles of human behavior. If you jumped off the roof of a tall building, your belief or disbelief in the law of gravity would not affect your impact on the ground. The same holds for the principles you will be using from this book. They WILL work if you use them. You can learn to believe in them after they work.

The change process is composed of four stages: (1) *accepting* the problem, (2) *learning* new skills to combat the problem, (3) *practicing* these skills to master the art of personal control, and (4) *maintaining* these skills for the rest of your life. Each of these stages may take months and will vary from person to person. The first stage, as I have already mentioned, is necessary for the other three to have any affect. I get many clients who have heard of our success and assume that I have some type of magic potion. They have not really accepted their problem. They want me to put the band-aid on them and make the hurt go away.

If practiced thoroughly and with the help of another person, the second stage should take about two months. The third stage may last another two to three months. Plan for the last stage to last about two to three years. This most important stage is the downfall of most therapy programs. The last chapter in the book is designed to give you some hints on how to continue your progress. Patience is most needed in this last phase. It also helps to have a strong support person giving you encouragement and comfort when you feel weak.

Importance of Support Systems

There is an inherent problem built in to learning skills out of a book. For example, very few people can learn calculus or algebra just by reading a book. It often takes the personal touch of a teacher or other individual—

offering suggestions, giving feedback, and otherwise interacting in the learning process. I highly recommend that the skills in this book be learned with the help of another person in your life. It may be helpful to go through the book with someone who shares your problem. Or you may want to turn to a close friend, someone who cares about you and is willing to spend time helping you work through the details of learning these skills. A family member or a professional therapist may also help you. If you are currently in therapy or considering contacting a therapist, find out if he or she would be willing to help you go through this book. The therapist can help you in learning these skills, supplementing them along the way with various other issues that may come up and are important for you to deal with.

Use of a support person. A support person is anyone who cares about you enough to help you through this difficult change period. Most of us become discouraged when attempting to learn something new and difficult. It is helpful to have someone near who can give us an "attaboy" now and then; to have a listener who can silently and lovingly hear our doubts and concerns. Knowing that someone cares can provide tremendous mental support.

If you have someone who can invest some time and emotional support in your journey, you are fortunate indeed. You can make the most progress by having this person read the book with you (at *your* speed). Sometimes support people identify a particular problem in their own life and use these skills for themselves. As you continue reading and learning together, your support person will be able to offer very practical support, because he or she will know the language of change and help spot the weak points in your learning.

If you don't have a support person (which is common with Deadly Dieters), you can still succeed. It will just be harder. You might want to look for a support group for eating disorders located in your area. If there is none, placing an announcement in your local newspaper may astound you with the response. If you would like some help in finding people in your area, write to me and I will send you information that might be helpful.

Using a therapist. If you are currently not seeing a therapist or are dissatisfied with the one you have, then you might consider finding one who can help you work through this book. If you are concerned about finding one you are comfortable with, you may want to skip to the last chapter and read the section called "Finding a Therapist." It is not necessary to find one who has had experience with eating disorders. It is much more important to find one who is willing to work for and with you. There is enough material in this book to give a competent therapist a good working outline for your change process. He or she can supplement this book with other information from the professional literature as you continue in therapy.

If you are unhappy with your present therapist, don't be afraid to voice your opinions. If your therapist really cares about you, he or she will encourage you to do what is right for you—even if that means going to another therapist.

Effective therapies seem to have some common elements. A study in 1979 by Zeiss and his colleagues in the *Journal of Consulting and Clinical Psychology* found four components present in therapies that worked. As you look for a good therapist, you might want to check to see if these are present.

1. Therapy should begin with an elaborated, well-planned rationale. You need to understand what the therapy is designed to do, the role of the therapist, your responsibility, and a reasonable approximation of the time it will take.

2. Therapy should provide you with training in skills that you can immediately and directly use in controlling your life.

3. Therapy should emphasize the independent use of these skills outside of your therapy sessions in order to give you the chance to master these skills on your own.

4. Therapy should encourage and support you to believe that your improvement is caused by your increased skillfulness, not the therapist's skillfulness.

How the Deadly Diet Kills

The subtitle of this book could be "How to keep anorexia or bulimia from killing you." As you probably already know, the mortality rate for eating disorders is anywhere from 8 to 15 percent, depending on which study is cited. *Medical attention is imperative while you are using this book*. You must find a physician who is willing to monitor your electrolytes and general health. Without proper medical supervision you are at far greater risk for developing serious health problems. Any specialist will do, as long as you believe that you are getting proper treatment. Our clinic has had the most success in referring our clients to family practice specialists, but you may have equal success with some other type of specialist.

The Deadly Diet can also kill you emotionally and socially. Most Deadly Dieters experience wild mood swings and feel as if their emotional life is eating them up inside. It is not uncommon for Deadly Dieters to find it difficult to express either anger or sadness. Many emotions get choked off, so that the person is an emotional cripple.

The Deadly Diet is also a very isolating experience. As the Deadly Diet continues, friends who were once sympathetic and useful begin to drift away. They become tired of the excuses and the seemingly callous disregard the Deadly Dieter has for her own personal welfare. Eventually, life becomes a cocoon-like existence with more and more distance developing between the Deadly Dieter and the needed support system. You can begin to see how deadly this diet really is: imminent physical danger, a shallow emotional existence, and social isolation. This combination leaves little of substance for an individual to call life.

Addictive Qualities of the Deadly Diet

The Deadly Diet is an expensive existence. The dieter often pays for eating very little with enormous financial bills from going to one specialist after another. When the problem becomes severe enough, it may mean hospitalization, which can run into thousands of dollars in a short period of time.

Binging may make this expense even worse. Clients who binge many times every day often liken the problem to a drug addiction. I believe it is in many ways the same thing. My definition of an addiction is a lifestyle in which something so consumes your life that you begin to make decisions damaging to your health, job, and personal relationships.

Some of my clients, very respectable in every other way, have turned to shoplifting and other antisocial behaviors in order to support their habit. Since they are basically decent human beings, you can imagine the tremendous guilt this adds to their already stressed-out life. With finances already strained to the limit, it is difficult to contemplate professional therapy which may cost $70 an hour or more. But in the long run, therapy is the cheapest alternative.

Like all addictions, this one is difficult to quit cold turkey. In spite of the stories you may have heard of some who may have conquered the problem this way, believing it may happen to you is pure wishful thinking. The odds are about the same as winning a national lottery.

The Behavioral Change Process

"How many psychologists does it take to change a light bulb?" goes the old joke. "Just one. But only if the light bulb really wants to change." There is truth in this humor, because mental health professionals cannot force lasting change on anyone. I have had clients who dropped out of therapy and returned later stating they were now ready to change. These clients have done extremely well. Those who come to me because someone else wants them to change or because they merely want to avoid the pain do not do so well. You can estimate your readiness to begin the change process by the following questionnaire.

Readiness for Change Questionnaire

☐ *Have you made a personal commitment to change?* This is the one private switch that nobody can turn on for you. Without this commitment, this book and all the therapies in the world are worthless.

☐ *Are you willing to learn proven techniques for change?* You don't have to believe in these techniques because they are based on scientific laws of human behavior. Your disbelief or skepticism will not hamper their effectiveness in your life.

☐ *Do you recognize that the change process will be unique for you?* Even if you know others who have conquered their eating disorder, you will have to personalize the process for yourself. Don't expect to follow in exactly the same footsteps as someone else.

☐ *Are you willing to be patient?* All of my clients want results yesterday. No matter how fast these techniques work, they will not be fast enough for you. You have taken a lifetime to develop these bad habits, and they will not disappear overnight.

☐ *Can you accept change as a lifelong learning process?* This is related to the previous question. No matter how much progress you make, there will always be room for improvement. My most successful clients continue their new skills for the rest of their lives. Those with the most severe setbacks stop using them when the pain level became imperceptible.

☐ *Can you stop waging battles you cannot win?* You need to learn how to distinguish between what is worth fighting for and what is not. Being happy and healthy is worth fighting for. Being thin is not. Sometimes letting go is the best way to deal with petty, culturally forced habits.

☐ *Are you willing to confront your problem with a positive attitude?* (Notice that I didn't ask you if you can do it yet.) Willingness implies being honest with yourself and daring to make mistakes.

☐ *Will you approach your change program one step at a time?* This means reading, studying, and mastering one chapter before moving on to the next one. It is tempting to expect some great mystery to be revealed in later chapters. Believe me, there is none. You can only build a house from the bottom up, not the top down.

☐ *Are you willing to take calculated risks?* This, too, is extremely difficult. Usually you take risks that are too big and guaranteed to fail. I am asking you to take risks calculated to structure you for success.

☐ *Do you expect to succeed?* There is nothing like a self-fulfilling prophecy to put you on one path or another. It's an old cliche: "If you expect to succeed, you will, if you expect to fail, you also will." Unfortunately, it is powerfully true.

☐ *Are you open to new information?* New information is a prerequisite for major change. Some of this information will be exciting, some of it painful. All of it will be beneficial in one way or another.

☐ *Will you build and use a support network?* You need to find out what type of support works best for you, who can provide the support, and how to go about getting it. Support is vital, even if it begins with just one person. Many have tried, but few have been successful in conquering the Deadly Diet by themselves.

If your answers to these questions honestly reflect a serious commitment on your part, then you are ready for one of the most exciting experiences in your life. You must also remember that there is a difference between learning a skill and mastering it. Although you may learn most of these skills in a matter of months, it may take years to master them. Every great musician continues to practice many hours per day, because he or she knows that mastery is a lifelong process. It is much better to continue mastering something than to think you have arrived and then realize that there is more to be done.

Don't be afraid to accept the fact that these skills will be needed for the rest of your life. Soon, with practice, they will become automatic and will require very little attention from you to be effective.

Before you seriously undertake your change program, you might want to list on a piece of paper any advantages and any disadvantages of getting rid of the Deadly Diet. Here are some suggestions:

Disadvantages

I may not get as much attention.
I will have to take risks.
Maybe it won't work.
I must face the unknown, the unpredictable.
It will cost me time and money.
It could be painful.
Others may not like the "new me."

Advantages

I can make new friends and improve current friendships.
I can live without guilt and depression.
I will feel better physically, emotionally, mentally.
I will be better off financially.
I will not waste so much time.
I will be rid of thinking of food all the time.
I will like myself more.

How To Sabotage Your Program

This book is intended to help you learn how to take care of your life by teaching you skills and showing you tools to accomplish this goal. If your real goal is to fool others into thinking you are serious about changing, when in fact you are not, then perhaps I can give you some help in accomplishing even this. To do this you must show those around you that you are reading this book and pretending to do the exercises. Outwardly, you will appear to be trying your best. Inwardly, you will do your best to sabotage the program. The following ten steps are guaranteed to help you subtly undermine the information in this book and the best efforts of therapists, friends, and family. (McMullin 1975)

1. Don't do any of the assignments when others are not around.

2. When they are around, do the assignments, but only halfheartedly; try not to concentrate too much on the material while you are doing it.

3. While you are working on one issue, spend a lot of time thinking of all the other issues that need your attention.

4. Deny any improvement, especially when it is small—wait for the big ones, even if it takes forever.

5. Refuse to believe that these skills will work for you, while encouraging others to use them.

6. Become convinced that you are different—these ideas and suggestions don't really apply to you.

7. Be sure to tell yourself every day that you are beyond help.

8. Halfway through the book, stop using it and look for a magic solution somewhere else.

9. Try to spend as much of your time as possible engaging in negative thinking—after all, no one can hear those thoughts.

10. Be sure you take total responsibility for your failures, but attribute any successes to luck.

Shortcomings of the Book

Many mental health professionals tend to degrade the value of self-help books. They complain that the claims made for them do not match the benefit they give the reader. Although there is some truth to this, it is important to acknowledge that many people have indeed been helped through such literature. For years, my own clients have benefited enormously through my recommendations of selected books that I thought might help them learn some important skill.

One shortcoming in this book is the incompleteness of our knowledge. The field of cognitive-behavioral therapy is very new. In spite of its tremendous power, our current techniques will be seen fifty years from now as primitive and inefficient. Another problem is the fact that few people learn best by reading a book. It is difficult because of the lack of interaction between the reader and author. I have found that no matter how well I describe something, some of my clients will not understand it until I say it another way. The reader of this book does not have the privilege of asking me questions. This is probably the most serious objection to self-help books in general.

On the other hand, I would not be writing this book if I did not think that there would be some benefit for those reading it. Many people have written to me asking for help with their eating disorder. They live in remote locations and have no access to experts in the field of eating disorders. I hope these people can gain some help from the suggestions in this book. Others have spent years learning about themselves in insight therapy and have experienced considerable personal growth. They wonder what to do next and ask for practical books to defeat the eating disorder. I hope this book will offer them valuable means for enhancing their learning. Therapists have also asked me for advice and information on how to work with eating disorders. I hope this book will increase their professional competence and allow them to further expand their skills.

The materials you will need to help in the learning process are:

spiral notebook
3-ring binder
2 sets of spiral-bound 3x5 index cards

The first will be used to keep all your written records and notes. When it fills up, start another one. Your progress can be closely estimated by how quickly you fill up your notebooks.

The binder will be used for your Success Journal and other copies of material that are important to you. There are now many resources for Deadly Dieters on the market. Keeping them in one place can be a valuable resource for you.

The spiral-bound index cards will become your Voice Fighting Kit. In the back you will have copies of the Understanding Your Emotions Chart and the Keyword Summary Chart. In the front you will put the Voice Fighting Decision Tree, the Personal Keywords Chart, and the Basic Voice Fighting Response.

1

The Epidemic of Affluence

Panic, handmaid of numbing fear.

—HOMER, *ILLIAD*, 850 B.C.

Suppose that you opened a newspaper tomorrow morning and read about a disease that was currently affecting 5 percent of the population. The story would be on page one, and it would describe great alarm on the part of public officials. Soon all forms of the media would be carrying daily stories on the problem. The Surgeon General would declare a national emergency. Some sections of the country might even be put under quarantine. People in every state would be in a state of panic lest the disease affect their family.

Yet, as you read these words, an epidemic is not happening in the United States which is not affecting just 5 or even 10 percent of the population. The epidemic I am speaking of probably affects 20 percent of females between the ages of thirteen and forty. The National Institute of Mental Health has recently estimated that five million American women suffer from an eating disorder. It is called the Deadly Diet. You probably know it by several of its more popular names: anorexia or bulimia.

The Extent of the Epidemic

Eating disorders are sweeping this country and are rampant on our junior high, high school, and college campuses. It is rare for any young female not to know of someone with an eating disorder. Although the statistics are still being gathered, it appears that at least one in five young women has a serious problem with eating and weight.

The Victims Are Female

The Deadly Diet basically appears to be a female problem. (Females also have a better chance of recovery than males.) Eating disorders are most prevalent in the middle to upper middle-class families—the so-called managerial-professional family. Currently the incidence is much lower in females from "blue-collar" families.

Estimates vary as to when this problem typically begins. The Deadly Diet can begin anywhere from the ages of ten to thirty. The peak age for the beginning of the Deadly Diet in females is between eleven and fifteen; the peak age for males is between fifteen and eighteen.

Although much of the information on the Deadly Diet says that it is a problem of teenage girls, our clinic has found that most of the people who come for therapy are in their twenties and thirties. This may be because younger people are generally less likely to seek professional help. Often it is the parent who brings the reluctant child to therapy. Adults who have left home and had to personally grapple with managing their lives usually tend to realize more clearly the need to seek help and make changes.

Is Our Culture To Blame ?

Even the most casual observer will notice that our culture places an extremely high value on women being thin. Although some people in the fashion business now claim that today's models are more filled out than those of a few years back, the evidence is difficult to see. An issue of *People* magazine in the winter of 1983 had a cover story on Karen Carpenter and the tragedy of her fight with the Deadly Diet. Yet the same issue had a lengthy story on one of America's top fashion models, with pictures showing a woman five feet, ten inches tall and weighing 110 pounds. The pictures of this model looked little different from those of Karen Carpenter in the few months before her death.

Our society evaluates and admires men for their vocation—what they accomplish and what they achieve. Women are usually evaluated by and accepted for how they look, regardless of what they do. A woman can be incredibly successful and still find that her beauty or lack of it will have more to do with her acceptance than what she is able to accomplish. From the time they are tiny children, most females are taught that beauty is the supreme objective in life. The peer pressure for girls in school to be skinny is often far greater than for boys to make a team. When it is spring, young girls all start thinking, "How am I going to look in my bathing suit? I better take a few more pounds off!"

Another reason that females are more prone to have this problem than males is that the personality characteristics underlying eating disorders are usually found in women. These characteristics, which will be discussed in detail later in this chapter, are probably passed down from generation to generation, from mother to daughter.

Dieting

It has been estimated that 90 percent of all women have dieted at one time or another, while 50 percent are on a diet at any one time. When asked to estimate weight, 90 percent of all women say they are overweight. This is an astonishing statistic. Most professionals consider a person healthy if they are within ten pounds of their preferred weight. Yet women have been forced to believe that they are overweight if they are not exactly at the expected body weight. How many women continue to believe they need to "take off just ten pounds"?

This perception is not limited to adults. Half of all girls start dieting before thirteen years of age. Amazingly, half of all eight- to nine-year-old girls are on a diet of some sort. The professional journal, *Pediatrics*, reported in 1988 that overweight children are subjected to ridicule by their peers at a very early age. Because of this, even thin girls as young as five or six are concerned about bodily image and are afraid of getting fat.

So why do girls become preoccupied with dieting? In 1987, Dr. Drewnowski of the University of Michigan School of Public Health identified three factors which contribute to early dieting: maturation, money, mother.

Girls become more acutely aware of their bodies at puberty. Dr. Drewnowski found a relationship between early maturation and early attempts at dieting. Girls who mature before the age of twelve tend to be heavier than average and therefore, he believes, may have an increased risk of developing an eating disorder.

Children of wealthy parents are inclined to be more anxious about body image and dieting than children in a lower socioeconomic status.

His study also found that about half of all dieting girls were encouraged to do so by their mothers. Although his study did not look at the influence of fathers and brothers, my experience has been that these family members can indirectly encourage dieting by making remarks about how girls look.

When Did It All Start?

Since we've become a wealthy nation and have the ability to eat whatever and whenever we want, we can now choose *not* to eat. Eating disorders are a problem of affluence and consequently a rare condition in societies where people are starving and don't know when they will eat again. Eating disorders only appear to be a problem in countries where people are well fed.

Are eating disorders more common today than they were years ago? Go back several hundred years and notice that the overweight women in the paintings of Ruben's time were regarded as models of beauty and charm. Before our contemporary emphasis on thinness as being next to godliness, people often saw obesity as a sign of health and prosperity.

Dr. Marianne Rosenzweig, a senior clinical psychologist at the University of Alabama's student health center in Tuscaloosa, compared female college students in the 1980s with students in the 1960s. She compared three factors regarding weight and three behaviors related to dieting.

Weight and Diet Trends of the 1980s and 1960s		
	1980	1960
Accurately assess body weight	42	55
Normal body weight	50	73
Underweight	31	13
Fasting	46	18
Pills	19	6
Vomiting	16	<1

You will notice that fewer students in the 80s were at their normal body weight or were able to correctly estimate their body weight. More of them, however, were underweight. In terms of using extreme measures for weight loss, the differences become more profound. Two-and-a-half times more students in the 80s fasted in order to lose or maintain weight. Three times as many used some form of diet pill, while vomiting jumped by a factor of sixteen.

Mass communication has brought with it an emphasis on making people fit into standard molds. In the flapper era women were seen as desirable if they had no curves but were shaped like that of a preadolescent girl. The advent of Twiggy firmly implanted in the public's mind that thin was where it was at. We must be careful not to minimize the role of television in the current epidemic of anorexia and bulimia. All of us are aware of the overwhelming influence that TV has had on the American public. The number of American homes with a TV set is currently 99.5 percent and the average on-time is six hours and 20 minutes per day. The average person watches 18,000 commercials each year. It is these commercials that tell the Deadly Dieter what to feel, how to look, and whom to want. Advertising executives depend on the ability of TV images to implant themselves in the mind, remain there, and cause people to imitate the characters and behavior in commercials. The Deadly Dieter seems to be particularly vulnerable to this influence.

How Is the Deadly Diet Different From Other Diets?

The Deadly Diet almost always starts off quite innocently as a normal diet. As the person takes off weight, she is praised and congratulated for having so much willpower. When the weight is taken off—and sometimes surprisingly quick—the person begins to think that maybe a few more pounds would be good insurance. Unfortunately, there is never enough "insurance." The pounds continue to slip away. And the person is caught in the unrelenting grip of the Deadly Diet.

From this point on, the Deadly Diet is very different from the average "diet." The average dieter may spend time thinking of weight and food, but with the Deadly Dieter these thoughts are obsessive. Some people have said to me, "Oh, wouldn't it be nice to have anorexia so that you wouldn't have to waste time thinking of your weight or what foods you eat." Nothing could be further from the truth. The Deadly Dieter thinks constantly of food. It is the first thing she thinks about when she awakens in the morning and the last thing she thinks about when she goes to bed at night. The time in between is continually filled with thoughts about food, calories, and weight.

The major difference between the regular dieter and the Deadly Dieter has to do with the issue of control. It is not, as some professionals have stated, that the Deadly Dieter is too much in control and needs to learn to let go. The Deadly Dieter is totally out of control. Even the "perfect" diet itself is out of control. The regular dieter is in control of the diet; the Deadly Dieter is controlled by the diet.

Types of Deadly Dieters

There are five basic types of Deadly Dieter. Although there are probably as many variations of these basic types as there are people in the world, all eating disorders fall into one of these types of Deadly Diets.

Fasting. This type of Deadly Dieter will often try to exist on only 500 calories per day, even though most nutritionists claim that a starvation diet is no lower than about 1200 calories a day. This person can get so distraught over any "extra" calories that she begins to see calories where there are virtually none. For example, I have had people tell me they are afraid to chew one piece of gum for fear they would take in too many calories. One Deadly Dieter was even afraid of the "calories" in a glass of water!

Binging. People who just binge, and consequently are obese, can also be called Deadly Dieters. They, too, are out of control. Their "diet" is constantly on their minds. It begins to kill them—not only in terms of their health, but also socially and personally. Although this book is not geared specifically for this type of Deadly Dieter, the skills and principles can easily be adapted to help the binge eater.

Binging-Purging. These people often begin their Deadly Diet as fasters. They soon learn that fasting also cuts them completely off from most social functions. In our society it is rare when people get together and don't have some type of food available. The solution to "being thin" and yet being able to eat is to get rid of your food after having eaten it. The most common form of purging is vomiting. A much less common method is the use of copious amounts of laxatives.

Fasting-Purging. This form of the Deadly Diet combines the worst of two other categories. The binge-purge individual may at least get some nutrition into her body and might even maintain a normal weight. The faster-purger will throw up her food or take laxatives even while subsisting on 500 calories a day. This devastating combination is what most often kills the Deadly Dieter.

Fasting-Binging. This is the most frustrating category, because the person will often go on a "normal" diet for as long as six months. After staying at a reasonable weight for a period of time, she will go on a binge, which can last another six months. During this time she will put on as much as 100 pounds. Most people involved in this person's life insist that she has the "willpower" to eat properly "if only she would make a commitment." Unfortunately, this attitude only confuses the issues. The person has the same problem with eating and weight as the other four types of Deadly Dieter—it just looks different on the outside.

Similarities & Differences of the Five Deadly Diets

Problems	BI	BI-FA	FA	BI-PU	FA-PU
Typical weight level	Normal to obese	Normal to obese	−15% normal weight	Normal ± 10%	−20% normal weight
Binging	Frequent	Episodic	No	Frequent	No
Preferred weight control method	Frequent restrictive diets	Episodic diets	Severe fasting exercise	Purging	Fasting-Purging Exercise
Body image distortion	No	No	Yes	Yes	Yes
Forbidden foods	Binges on them	Not applicable	Avoids them	Will binge if able to purge	Avoids and purges
Emotion after eating	Relief	Relief or anxiety	Extreme anxiety	Moderate anxiety	Moderate to severe anxiety
Eating influenced by moods	Yes	Yes	Yes	Yes	Yes
Presence of secondary psycho-pathology	Moderate	Moderate	Severe	Moderate to severe	Severe to extreme

BI = Binging; BI-FA = Binging-Fasting; FA = Fasting; BI-PU = Binging-Purging; FA-PU = Fasting-Purging

For our purposes in this book, all five types of Deadly Dieter will be treated as similar. They all share the same problem—the underlying, common denominator of being out of control. EATING IS NOT THE ISSUE! The issue is the lack of control in all areas: physiological, emotional, mental, and behavioral.

The chart on the previous page compares some of the similarities and differences of the five Deadly Diets. The chart looks at: typical weight levels, binging, the typical method used for weight control, amount of distorted body image, how forbidden foods are dealt with, emotions related to eating, and the presence of other psychological problems.

Definition of the Deadly Diet

The mental health community has defined two of the five types of Deadly Diet: anorexia and bulimia. The definitions have been very carefully constructed and are good guidelines for determining if you have either disorder.

The "official" definition of anorexia nervosa consists of five components:

1. An intense fear of becoming obese, which does not diminish as weight loss progresses

2. Disturbance of body image, or claiming to "feel fat" even when emaciated

3. Weight loss of at least 25 percent of original body weight

4. Refusal to maintain body weight over a normal weight for age and height

5. No known physical illness that would account for the weight loss

The definition for bulimia (from the Greek words meaning "animal hunger") is also composed of five parts:

1. Recurrent episodes of binge eating

2. Awareness that the eating pattern is abnormal and fear of not being able to stop eating voluntarily

3. Depressed mood and self-deprecating thoughts following eating binges

4. The bulimic episodes are not due to anorexia or any other known physical disorder

5. At least three of the following conditions: (a) consumption of high-caloric, easily digested food during a binge; (b) unconspicuous eating during a binge; (c) termination of such episodes by abdominal pain,

sleep, social interruption, or self-induced vomiting; (d) repeated attempts to lose weight by severely restricted diets, self-induced vomiting, or use of cathartics or diuretics; (e) frequent weight fluctuations greater than ten pounds due to alternating binges and fasts

Physical Problems

In addition to the symptoms above, anorexia and bulimia can also be accompanied by medical side effects. For anorexia, some of these symptoms may include feeling cold even in hot weather, fatigue and lack of energy, loss of menstruation, skin problems, inability to sweat, chilblains, swelling in the face, dehydration, and even gangrene of the fingertips.

Some of the physical symptoms associated with bulimia include sweating, breathlessness, rapid heartbeat, hot flashes, and many of the symptoms associated with anorexia listed above.

But perhaps the most dangerous physical result of any form of the Deadly Diet is the potential for an electrolyte imbalance. This is often discovered as a low potassium level. Low potassium is one of the most common causes of nocturnal cardiac arrest, and many of the deaths associated with the Deadly Diet are the result of cardiac arrest. Since an electrolyte imbalance can literally be a matter of life and death, it is of the utmost importance for anyone with an eating disorder to be under the care of a knowledgeable physician.

For three types of Deadly Diet—Fasting, Fasting-Purging, and Fasting-Binging—starvation is one of the key ingredients. Most people who fast think 1000 calories is the magic number to avoid. Deadly Dieters often go for half of that. In reality, most nutritionists and dieticians promote 1200 calories as the starvation cut-off.

The problem with fasting is that it dramatically decreases glycogen, fats, and proteins in the body. These elements are vital in the production of glucose, which is the basic energy source for all the body's systems. The body needs energy for its activities including organ function, not just physical exercise. To rob the energy storage areas is similar to living off the principal, rather than the interest, in your savings. If the principal (fat) is sufficient, you can live for a long time. Once the principal is gone, however, the interest is the only thing left and the process of self-destruction is inevitable. When a person decreases her energy input (starvation), the body goes through three fairly well-defined stages.

Stage one begins immediately. The day a person begins fasting the carbohydrate stores in the body begin to become depleted. Low glucose levels trigger a response in the body which makes the pancreas begin to secrete glucagon in the liver which is then released into the body as glucose. This operation allows the body to continue functioning to keep the energy levels at needed efficiency.

While this mechanism for replacing lost energy in the body is occurring, other events are taking place which are identified as the second stage of starvation. A special type of body fat, lipids, are the primary energy source for most body cells. The liver is one of the major organs for metabolizing fatty acids and when it does the ketone bodies are produced in large quantities and transported to body and brain cells. Unfortunately, these cells can only use a finite amount of ketones, so the excess spills over into the blood and is known as a condition called ketosis. The excessive ketones in the blood result in a decrease in the pH of the blood. Eventually a problem called metabolic acidosis develops which causes depression of the central nervous system and can eventually lead to coma. The length of this second stage depends on the amount of stored body fat.

When the fat stores are depleted, the third stage begins. This causes the proteins, which are needed to maintain cellular functioning, to break down as an energy source. When protein stores are depleted to about one-half their normal level, death usually results within 24 hours.

Nutrition

Many of my clients appear to be quite knowledgeable in nutrition, some even being nurses, registered dieticians, and nutritionists. In a sponsored study which appeared in the *International Journal of Eating Disorders* sixty-eight questions concerning nutrition were presented to people with eating disorders and people with normal eating habits. The results showed that Deadly Dieters knew more about nutrition in the areas of macronutrients, roughage, and calories. Both groups were about equally informed regarding questions of vitamins. The researchers concluded that people with eating disorders know how to eat well and care for their bodies. The problem is that they are unable to use information properly for reasons you will discover later in this book.

At the University of Michigan, Dr. Dean Krahn found that people with eating disorders consumed high levels of caffeine. He defined high daily caffeine intake as: fifteen cups of tea, or eight cups of coffee, or sixteen 12-ounce sodas. His study seemed to indicate that the excessive caffeine might even worsen the behaviors of the Deadly Diet, such as binge eating and vomiting.

As already mentioned, it is very difficult for your body to get the nutrients it needs to maintain good health when you consume fewer than 1000 calories a day. To be sure you get all the nutrition your body requires, eat a diet that includes servings from each of the basic food groups. Rather than eliminating certain food groups or concentrating on just one or two food groups, it is better to keep a variety of foods in your diet but change the portion size. Your body also desperately needs fats in your

Eating Suggestions for
Those With Bulimia

- Avoid "trigger foods" (those you associate with a binge) at first. These can be reintroduced later in your treatment. Instead, eat a nutrient-dense replacement that has some of the same pleasant characteristics.

- Eat three planned meals a day, rather than smaller, more frequent meals—this will help you to avoid binges.

- Eat foods that require the use of utensils, rather than eating finger foods. This will slow eating time and help increase meal satisfaction.

- Include generous portions of carbohydrate-containing foods.

- Include low-calorie items in each meal, such as vegetables, broth-based soup, salad, and/or fruit, to prolong the mealtime.

- Include adequate fat, which slows the emptying of food from the stomach to increase meal satisfaction.

- Eat a variety of foods at each meal.

- Eat all meals and snacks sitting down.

- Include hot or warm foods, rather than eating just cold or room-temperature foods.

- Plan meals ahead, using a food diary.

- Use foods that are naturally divided into portions, such as one potato (rather than rice or pasta); 4- and 8-ounce containers of yogurt, ice cream, or cottage cheese; precut steaks or chicken parts; and frozen dinners and entrees.

diet. As you saw above, fats are essential for maintaining proper body functioning. Rather than eliminating them from your foods, you would be wiser to increase physical activity to help control body fat.

Since you will not be able to significantly change your eating patterns until you have mastered the techniques in this book, I have included some eating suggestions which can help tide you over and contribute to good health until you discard your Deadly Diet. These suggestions have

Eating Suggestions for Those With Anorexia Nervosa

- Eat small frequent meals to help reduce bloating.

- Begin to introduce fat into your diet, because fat is needed as a necessary ingredient of good health.

- Eat foods cold or at room temperature to decrease early feelings of fullness.

- Eat finger foods, or snacks.

- Eat high-fiber foods to encourage good bowel habits.

- Limit fruits and vegetables because the soluble fiber they contain slows the emptying of food from the stomach and may make you feel bloated.

- Limit caffeine intake because it may interfere with normal appetite patterns.

- Take a multivitamin-multimineral supplement, as recommended by your physician or nutrition counselor.

been adapted from the pamphlet, *Nutrition and Eating Disorders*, by Patterson, Whelan, Rock & Lyon, 1989.

Exercise

How much energy you dissipate during exercise is determined by your age, sex, height, weight, basal metabolic rate, dietary history, and level of physical activity. It is a common illusion among Deadly Dieters that you only burn energy when you are active. The basal metabolic rate is the amount of energy that your body uses when at rest. As you increase physical activity, you increase your basal metabolic rate and your lean tissue mass (muscle).

The best way to measure your basal metabolic rate, determine how many calories you need daily, and the amount of healthy exercise you need is to have yourself water-weighed by a reputable organization. By measuring your weight under water and checking your lung capacity, you can calculate how to be healthy. If you would like to approximate how many calories you need per day, complete the following steps:

Calculating Calories Needed

1. Calculate estimated ideal body weight: _____

   Men: 106 pounds for the first five feet of height plus 6 pounds for each additional inch
   Women: 100 pounds for the first five feet of height plus 5 pounds for each additional inch

2. Adjust your ideal body weight based on your frame size: _____

   Add 10% if you have a larger-than-average frame size
   Subtract 10% if you have a smaller-than-average frame size
   (Keep in mind that this is just an estimation)

3. Daily calorie expenditure: _____calories

   If sedentary: Ideal body weight x 13
   If moderately active: Ideal body weight x 15
   If active: Ideal body weight x 17
   If very active: Ideal body weight x 19

Gail

Gail was an above average teenager who was looked up to by her friends, classmates, and teachers. She came from a good home with loving parents who were concerned about their children but did not push them into any particular direction either academically or vocationally. Gail's father was a professional man, her mother was college educated and very active in community affairs. Both parents had an honest concern for people and had brought up Gail and her younger sister to respect people and to be sensitive and kind to those less fortunate than themselves.

Although she had a good relationship with both her mother and father, Gail began to exert her independence like most other normal teenagers when she was about fourteen. However, none of her adolescent mini-rebellions could have been considered extraordinary by any reasonable standards. Her developmental history was quite normal, and in all respects her family life was as good as anyone could wish for.

As with most girls, in high school Gail became very conscious of and sensitive about her weight. She admitted that this concern was mostly the result of what she saw in magazines and on television and what she heard from her girlfriends. One day a boy whom she secretly admired made a joking remark about her weight. Although she was somewhat hurt by the comment, she soon forgot it.

It wasn't long after that she and a friend decided to go on a diet "to lose a couple of pounds" before bikini weather rolled around. They both picked a sensible plan based on balanced nutrition and in three weeks both had lost 5 pounds.

Except that Gail decided this was not enough and thought she needed to try for a couple more pounds off. Her girlfriend did not agree and told Gail she looked fine. This was the beginning of the Deadly Diet for Gail, as she eventually dropped from 130 pounds on a five-foot-six-inch frame to 95 pounds. By this time her friends and family were becoming worried. Gail would skip breakfast and lunch and just pick at her food during dinner. Her daily caloric intake averaged about 500 calories. Even this sometimes felt like too much for her. She knew that she had become obsessed with food, had a phobic fear of gaining weight, and yet could do nothing about it.

When confronted by family and friends about her weight, she typically became defensive and denied having a problem, yet deep within she knew something was drastically wrong. She felt fearful, depressed, and guilty much of her waking hours. Often she thought that she might be going crazy. It was not until she was able to talk with other girls her age who were recovering from the Deadly Diet that she was able to admit she needed help in dealing with the problem.

Sally

Sally's bulimia ironically had started as anorexia when she was in her late teens. She had never really looked emaciated because she had learned from some friends that you can control your weight by throwing up your food right after eating. When she heard this, it was as if a burden had been lifted from her shoulders. Not only could she begin eating again, but she could also eat as much of the "forbidden" foods as she wanted to by just getting rid of it. When her family started to notice she was eating more, they were pleased. It seemed to them that she became a new person almost overnight.

Soon after Sally went away to college, and much to her surprise she discovered that many of the women in the dorm were also vomiting their food after eating. Sometimes she would worry about her "binge and barf" behavior and feel depressed or guilty. Other times, she would rationalize it by thinking that if so many other people were doing it, it couldn't be that bad. And it really was helping her maintain her weight. Through the years she would go through cycles in which the Deadly Diet would increase and decrease in frequency from several times a week to several times a day. These cycles would often be related to her various mood swings. When she was in her late thirties, with a good husband and two teenage children, she decided to go back to work. Although she enjoyed her job, when its pressures became more intense she found that the Deadly Diet became worse. Finally one day her husband caught her throwing up in the bathroom. When he realized that it was not because she was sick, his reaction threatened to tear their marriage apart. Sally began to realize that it was about time she did something about her problem, and she began to look for professional help.

Deadly Dieter Profile

Our clinic has developed a profile that seems to fit many of the people who come to us for treatment. It should help you see the similarities between yourself and others who have been captured by the Deadly Diet. Complete the following survey and then read carefully the explanation of each profile characteristic.

Eating Disorder Profile

	Yes	No
1. Are you a worrier?	☐	☐
2. Are you a perfectionist?	☐	☐
3. Do you have a lot of stress in your life?	☐	☐
4. Do you ever feel like you're losing control?	☐	☐
5. Do you get nervous when your daily routine is upset?	☐	☐
6. Have you ever had a panic attack?	☐	☐
7. Do you talk to yourself a lot?	☐	☐
8. Do you have a poor self-image?	☐	☐
9. Are you ever concerned about what others think?	☐	☐

10. Which of the following emotions do you experience and how often?

	Never	Sometimes	Frequently
Depression	☐	☐	☐
Guilt	☐	☐	☐
Helplessness	☐	☐	☐
Resentment	☐	☐	☐
Unhealthy Anxiety	☐	☐	☐
Unreasonable Fear	☐	☐	☐

Explanation of the Profile

Worry. Worry is a Deadly Diet characteristic that has escaped professional attention. Yet every client I have seen at the clinic has been a worrier: a constant, chronic, unbelievable worrier. This is not your everyday variety of worry. When this kind of worrier isn't worried, she worries because she's not worrying. When friends are around, nobody else has to worry because the Deadly Dieter worries for everybody. Most clients say to me, "I don't remember a time in my life when I didn't worry. I can remember being four years old and worrying about something."

One of my clients remembered an incident that happened when she was seven years old. An earthquake, which occurred 900 miles from where she lived, caused her to worry about earthquakes for an entire year. Even when she was finally shown on a map how far away it had been, she still continued to worry. In fact, many Deadly Dieters grow up thinking that worry is the norm. When they become adults and realize that nobody else worries like they do, they begin to worry about being so different.

Perfectionism. Perfectionism does not mean that you always have a clean house or room all the time. Rather, it is a method of making decisions that stresses extreme options. As a perfectionist, when you have a task to do, you will either try to do it flawlessly or not at all. There is no middle ground. Few Deadly Dieters are full-time perfectionists, but most usually think that in one or two areas of their life things have to be "just so." Often these areas of perfectionism are associated with an *overall* sense of self-worth. By not allowing mistakes in these few areas, perfectionists can feel good about themselves in general and stay insulated from failures and mistakes in other areas. One woman who came to our clinic was admired by others for being able to get so many things done in a day and still do them so well. During therapy she came to realize this quality was really a manifestation of her wanting to be perfect in everything she did. Unfortunately, the perfectionism was controlling and ruining her life.

Stress. Many of my clients seem to have stress that never goes away. Never—despite yoga, biofeedback, or even hypnosis. In fact, their stress can be so common they learn to live with it and accept it as normal. Sometimes when I ask the question, "Do you have a lot of stress?" they will respond, "No, I don't think I do." With further questioning I find out that they suffer enormous amounts of stress and believe it is an inevitable part of their life. They may have headaches, insomnia, fatigue, or loss of concentration.

Control. The issue of control is just beginning to be recognized in psychology as a significant part of human behavior. Many of the therapists who first worked with the Deadly Diet thought that their clients were "too much in control." Even today, some therapists who work with Deadly Dieters think that the eating disorder is deliberately used to "control" or manipulate or use other people. This is the exact opposite of what is really happening. Deadly Dieters are hopelessly out of control; the last thing in the world they are able to control is their eating behavior. The central problem is that the eating controls them. Many of my clients will tell me, "Nobody really understands me when I tell them I feel out of control. They think I'm nuts, and sometimes I begin to wonder if maybe I really am going crazy."

Inflexibility. Many Deadly Dieters find themselves mentally planning their days and nights compulsively around food. When events occur that upset these plans, they get terribly nervous and irritable. It is often difficult for them to act spontaneously. They dread the unexpected for fear that something will happen to make them lose further control. Their ritualistic behavior is a means of trying to keep control of their life. One anoretic man told me that the moment he woke up in the morning he would begin thinking about food. He would mentally plan out his day— every event revolved around food and his avoidance of it. If he had to go some place where there might be food, he creatively figured out how to not get involved in the event. When he went to bed at night he knew that sleep was only a temporary relief from the same process, which would begin all over again the next morning.

Panic attacks. A panic attack is a stress reaction of terrifying proportions. About one-third of Deadly Dieters report having them. Most find that words are inadequate to describe the subjective reaction they have to a panic attack. One client put it this way: "It feels like you're going to die, you know you're not, but you wish you would." Deadly Dieters who have panic attacks find food even more disruptive than other Deadly Dieters.

Internal dialogue. Some of my clients are not initially aware of the mental battle that takes place continuously within their minds, but many do report the feeling of a constant debate going on inside their head. Others report no such internal conversations. With these individuals, the dialogue is so pervasive they are just not aware of it. One client told me that this internal dialogue "went on continually and never stopped," even when she tried hard to force herself to think of other things.

Self-image. When asked if they have a poor self-image, about nine out of ten Deadly Dieters will answer yes. I find this quite ironic, because they tend to have qualities admired by most people. They are often kind, considerate, personable, likable, bright, and creative. Deadly Dieters are very often looked up to and admired by others, and their poor self-image does not fit their high level of achievement. Although some professional therapists still see the Deadly Dieter as manipulative and generally un-successful in life, this is simply not true!

Evaluation by others. Constant attention to what others think can become so habitual and obsessive that it often turns into a mental dis-tortion called mind reading—"knowing" what others are thinking with-out any indication or confirmation from the other person. Of course, these evaluations *always* turn out to be negative. Even after receiving a com-pliment, one of my clients thought to herself, "They didn't really mean that. They just said it to be nice."

Destructive emotions. Although not all Deadly Dieters experi-ence all six destructive emotions all of the time, these emotions still tend to be significant factors in the life of the Deadly Dieter. In fact, feelings such as depression are so common that many therapists misdiagnose the Deadly Diet as a depressive disorder. A middle-aged woman told that she had been to three psychiatrists and all of them had told her she was probably depressed and going through her mid-life crisis. They gave her pills to make her feel better. One therapist was so insistent that these emotions were the primary diagnosis that my client never mentioned her eating disorder to him again, even though she continued seeing this ther-apist for another year.

If, after reading the descriptions of the Deadly Dieter Profile, you have concluded that your eating behavior (or diet, if you prefer) may be controlling you rather than you controlling it, then this book may be for you. It is designed to help you, step by step, to a life of freedom, a life that can be personally satisfactory and growing. This book will not show you how to live a life with no problems. Everybody has problems and will always have them. Having problems is not the issue; the issue is how you cope with them. This book will teach you how to cope effec-tively with your Deadly Diet.

Professional Approaches to the Deadly Diet

There are currently four major approaches to the understanding and treat-ment of the Deadly Diet. The first of these methods goes back to the beginnings of mental health. The last one is relatively new and is so pow-erful that it is fast becoming the main treatment alternative of successful therapists.

TREATMENT   Approaches :

"If We Could Only Find Out Why You Do This"

I

The first effort to explain and understand eating disorders began with the theories of Sigmund Freud. He postulated a number of drives and structures brewing deep within the mind that *force* individuals to behave in various ways. His attempts to alleviate mental illness were often unsuccessful, yet thousands of therapists are still trying to use these ideas to help Deadly Dieters. One of the earliest theories assumed that the problem was some type of "organ system vulnerability." In other words, it was believed there was a biological reason for the problem. Since no evidence of this was found, the hypothesis was eventually discarded. Some current researchers have resurrected the idea, but there is still confusion as to which comes first—the medical condition or the Deadly Diet. The idea that the Deadly Diet has some type of symbolic meaning representing a deeper cause is also still accepted by some therapists today. Some of the various explanations for the Deadly Diet have been "a form of psychosomatic disturbance," "a wish for a father-penis-baby," "a form of schizophrenia," "a rejection of a wish to be pregnant," "an attempt to reestablish the mother-child unity," "a displacement of sexual fears," "a deep-seated fear of a nourished body," and "an ego-disorganization along the lines of schizophrenic despair."

Unfortunately, most psychological approaches that try to treat human problems through the analysis of symbolic processes are more concerned with understanding "why" a person has the Deadly Diet than finding specific methods to treat the problem. Still more unfortunately, they often do more harm than good to the Deadly Dieter seeking treatment.

"Mom and Dad Are To Blame"

This method, which was at its peak in the 1970s, is called the Family Systems approach. It attempts to understand the Deadly Diet as a result of conflicts within the family structure. In other words, "as the family goes, so goes the Deadly Diet." As a girl reaches adolescence, her attempts to define her identity and independence apart from her family cause her to feel guilty and ungrateful. This internal struggle between independence and dependence violates her internal image of herself as a "good girl." Rather than be involved in open warfare with her parents, she concentrates her attention on something more manageable—her weight.

The Deadly Diet is seen as a part of an overall power struggle between the girl and her parents in which the girl has the ultimate power—the power of death. The entire procedure of the family systems approach is brought to bear on this "dysfunctional family" and the Deadly Diet is treated by dealing with communication patterns, overprotection, conflict avoidance, and coping behaviors. In fact, many family therapists prefer to deal with the "psychosomatic family" rather than just with the Deadly Dieter. Some of the more radical family therapists will not even see a Deadly Dieter unless it is done within the context of the family.

Although many of these therapists claim a "success rate" of over 85 percent, this approach has two serious flaws in its ability to deal effectively with Deadly Diets. The first is that many young girls with Deadly Diets come from very normal families. It would be unjust to classify these families as dysfunctional. Many times these "dysfunctional families" are so labeled because of circular thinking (a common problem in mental health). The thinking goes something like this: If asked why a girl uses the Deadly Diet, the therapist answers, "Because she is living in a dysfunctional family." "How do you know the family is dysfunctional?" is the next question. Answer: "Because the girl is a Deadly Dieter."

The second major flaw in this approach is related to newer data that shows that Deadly Diets are not the exclusive domain of young girls. More and more older women are appearing in clinics for the treatment of the Deadly Diet. In our clinic, only about 25 percent of Deadly Diet clients are girls younger than twenty. Many are in their twenties and thirties, with a few even in their forties. Most of these clients do not live in the home, nor do they have frequent contact with their families.

"A Product of the Environment"

A third approach to the treatment of Deadly Diets is probably the most effective of the three—under very limited conditions. The behavioral approach treats the Deadly Diet as the product of the environment. It is a "learned" condition which can be "unlearned" by reshaping the person's environment so that the individual can use better coping behaviors. This has become the treatment of choice in institutional settings where the staff can have total control over the Deadly Dieter's environment.

Through a series of rewards and punishments, often dramatic results are obtained which are inconceivable through other more insight-oriented approaches. Unfortunately, the effectiveness of this treatment is diminished by its failure to transfer to other, less controlled environments. When the Deadly Dieter leaves the institutional setting, the old environmental triggers are still around, and the Deadly Diet tends to come back. This method is further hampered because, to the person with the Deadly Diet, no reinforcement may be capable of counteracting the reinforcement offered by the avoidance of food or an all-out binge.

"You Are What You Think"

This approach appears to have the most promise for working with the Deadly Dieter. Along the way, it teaches the Deadly Dieter:

DISCUSS

- to accept personal responsibility for his or her actions
- to be a less-than-perfect person
- to effectively and independently solve personal problems
- to correct mental distortions about weight
- to be a growing and maturing individual
- to take risks and be vulnerable to life
- to identify his or her needs and get them met
- to take complete control of his or her life

Eating Disorders as Phobias

Originally, very few people working with Deadly Diet clients noticed the similarity to phobic individuals. Since the early 70s there have been more people who have observed how Deadly Diets tend to be phobic in nature. In 1983 a group of researchers in British Columbia, Canada, did a comparative study between Deadly Dieters, phobics, and people with obsessive-compulsive problems. Although this study concluded that Deadly Diets were more like an obsessive-compulsive disorder, it was apparent from the discussion of what phobias were like that the researchers did not really understand the thoughts and feelings of the person suffering from a severe phobia.

The "official" definition of a phobia is "a persistent, irrational fear of, and compelling desire to avoid, an object or situation." The person using the Deadly Diet is also controlled by an irrational, overwhelming, runaway fear—that of getting fat! If you ask a Deadly Dieter what she fears most in life, she will say, "gaining weight" or "getting fat," even though "fat" may mean only one-half pound. The person with a phobia avoids things that bring on unhealthy anxiety; likewise, the Deadly Dieter avoids things related to food that can bring on extreme anxiety. These anxieties are pervasive and tend to intrude into the person's life on a regular basis.

The similarities between the Deadly Dieter and the person with a severe phobia fall into four categories: mental distortions, high stress levels, destructive emotions, and rituals (avoidance behaviors).

Mental distortions. One of the foremost features common to both problems is the intense worry that characterizes the person's daily thought life. Both Deadly Diets and phobias involve destructive self-statements such as the "what ifs," "shoulds," and the use of absolutist words such as "never" and "always." Both groups of people are intensely worried about what other people think of them. In fact, this one thought is often the driving force behind avoidance behaviors. Perfectionism in phobics and Deadly Dieters results from the mistaken idea that a person's worth is equal to his or her behavior. Therefore, the person cannot allow herself to make a mistake for fear of being proven worthless. Another chronic worry is the conviction of poor self-image. The irony is that while the person is convinced that she is worthless, she compulsively strives to behave "perfectly" in order that others will not see her total imperfection.

High stress. Extreme levels of stress are also common for both Deadly Dieters and people with phobias. The evidence for this stress is often seen in headaches, insomnia, hyperventilation, or panic attacks. The stress makes it difficult for the person with a phobia or Deadly Diet to learn even the most basic skills for working on her problems. Ironically, few people with these problems have tried to do anything about the stress—other than, perhaps, exercise—and some don't even know what techniques are available for the reduction of stress. Some of the more common methods people have tried for dealing with stress are medication, biofeedback, yoga, and meditation. Many times these techniques work for a while and then lose their effectiveness because the person stops practicing the skills.

Ask about

Destructive emotions. The third similarity between phobias and eating disorders is the presence of destructive emotions. What was pointed out earlier about misdiagnosing depression for the Deadly Diet holds equally for phobias. Many people with phobias have been classified as neurotic, hysterical, depressed, and even "schizoid." In addition to depression, almost all people with phobias and Deadly Diets tend to feel guilty a great portion of the time. They tend to take on the unrealistic expectations of others and society in general. A feeling of helplessness and being trapped is also very common. This feeling occurs when the person's options begin to narrow down so that very few choices are left for everyday decisions. Anxiety and fear are also destructive emotions common to both phobias and Deadly Diets. In fact, all of these emotions are so common that when a Deadly Dieter and a person with a phobia meet for the first time and get beyond their behavioral differences, they are amazed at how similar their problems tend to be. When we combine both populations into a treatment group, the Deadly Dieter can empathize with those who have phobias, while those with phobias can understand what happens internally to those suffering from the Deadly Diet.

Freedom

Rituals. The final similarity is the existence of ritualistic coping behaviors. These usually involve some type of situational avoidance. In the case of the Deadly Dieter it means avoiding the effects of food on her body. The faster simply doesn't put much in, while the binger-purger tries to take it back out as fast as she puts it in. The phobic will often avoid a broader range of situations: high places, freeways, elevators, large crowds, certain animals or insects. It is not uncommon, however, for both groups of people to avoid many social situations. If the problem has continued for any length of time, social avoidance can be common for both groups of people.

The Control Cycle

As has been stated, being out of control is THE major feature of the Deadly Diet. For some, the feeling of lack of control is just concerned with eating and weight control. For others, it seems that everything in their life is out of control.

Every Deadly Diet consists of five basic components that together comprise the Control Cycle. They are: (1) environmental triggers, (2) destructive thoughts, (3) high stress, (4) ineffective coping behaviors, and (5) destructive emotions. These are interrelated to one another as illustrated in the diagram on the next page.

Situation. The situation refers to anything out there that triggers the Control Cycle. Of course, for the Deadly Dieter the trigger is usually something to do with food. Eating is a large part of our culture that is built into our social habits, and there are a lot of triggers in life for the Deadly Dieter. How many times have you socialized with someone and not had something to eat or drink? These external triggers set off characteristic worries, destructive self-statements, doubts, and self-attacks.

Thoughts. The worry, the kicking of self, the old painful memories that suddenly erupt are a habit that feels like a totally independent entity. It seems independent because people with Deadly Diets tend to be quite intelligent and "know" that most of the worries and irrational thoughts are meaningless. Many people have told me that they wished they didn't worry so much but that they "just can't help it." To even dream of a life without worry is to engage in a fantasy of immense proportions. The chronic worry, in turn, is responsible for two more things happening: stress and destructive emotions.

Stress. You will notice on the diagram that stress is internally generated, not externally generated. In other words, stress comes about because of what you think, not because of what is happening to you. We know this to be true because some people can be relaxed and calm in the most distressing circumstances, while others can be coming apart at the seams in the mildest situations. Remember that stress is not an emotion, but a physiological event that can influence the type of behaviors we use to cope with life.

Emotions. The worry also causes one or more destructive emotions. These emotions in turn add more stress to the body. But they also compel a person to engage in some type of coping behavior to counteract the feelings of unpleasant emotions and high stress.

Behavior. When you are feeling highly emotional and your body is feeling stressed, you are generally in a high discomfort zone. This off-balance experience motivates you to do something in order to "feel better." What you eventually do is get caught in ritualistic behaviors. For example, when you feel bored, your reflex reaction might be to binge; when you have a stress headache, you might be even less likely to eat even your self-imposed 500 calorie limit. Avoidance behavior is one of the most common rituals. Not eating is an obvious example of avoidance for the faster. The binger-purger is often involved in a double-avoidance

Control Cycle

Situation

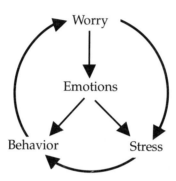

ritual. She may eat to avoid "feeling bad" and then purge herself in order to avoid feeling guilty for binging.

Often avoidance becomes an entire lifestyle. The person will avoid anything that presents a conflict, anything that can cause pain. A psychologist from Canada has coined the phrase "discomfort dodging" to describe this experience. Over a period of time, people who tend to avoid life's friction become passive, nonassertive persons, and this avoidance in turn causes them to worry even more.

The problem with Deadly Diets is not primarily the behavior, even though the behavior is what tells others that something is wrong. The problem illustrated by the Control Cycle is that ritual behaviors can bring the person right back to the top of the cycle: more worry, and on around the cycle in a never-ending pattern. For example, after a person has avoided food or binged and purged, she will often engage in a series of destructive evaluations of herself that will continue the cycle indefinitely.

When shown this cycle, people with Deadly Diets say, "That is exactly how I feel. I feel like I am going around in circles, like my life is a merry-go-round and I can't get off." The situation triggers worry, worry triggers stress and destructive emotions, the emotions add to the stress, and then the person spends considerable time ineffectively coping with the problem—which then starts all over again.

Example

Joan had been struggling with bulimia for over five years and had found herself caught up in this vicious cycle of out-of-controllness. Even though she could go for a couple of weeks at a time without binging, when it did happen she felt as if she had absolutely no control of what was taking place. The situational triggers for Joan often revolved around her mother, who tended to call her several times a day from the other side of town and inquire into the private affairs of her family. After some of these conversations, she became very upset but said nothing to her mother. Her husband was finally tired of hearing about the problem and had told her to be more assertive with her mother. When the control cycle was finally analyzed it was found that the telephone conversations with her mother triggered several thematic thoughts: "I resent my mother implying that I don't know how to run my family. But if I were to say anything to her, she would get upset and I would feel guilty. It is sure unfair that my mother and I cannot have a good relationship." These thoughts often were stressful enough to bring on a severe headache, either by itself or along with the feelings of depression, guilt, and helplessness. When either of these things occurred, she would secretly binge and vomit her food. When this ritual was completed, she would start putting herself down for what she had just done and telling herself that she should know better. This in turn triggered more guilt and stress. Joan was now caught up in the vicious out-of-control cycle.

Irwin had been struggling with anorexia for over ten years and had come to a point in his life where he was sick and tired of what was happening to him. Before coming to the clinic, he would find that the mere sight of food (trigger) would begin all types of doomsday messages (worry). Some of these included: "What if I started to eat and lost control. I would blow up like a blimp and that would be a tragedy. All of these feelings within are really dangerous—they could really hurt me." These destructive thoughts made him hyperventilate (stress) and feel anxiety and fear (destructive emotions). Together these components would get him to avoid food for as long as possible (behavior). The avoidance would cause him to worry about his health and overall general lack of happiness and fulfillment.

Three Basic Skills

The endless nature of the Control Cycle is what makes Deadly Diets so terrifying. No matter what you do, you wind up in the same place. When you get caught in this vicious cycle, you spend all your energy going around in circles. Life becomes a treadmill, and you live it like a hamster running on a wheel that never goes anywhere.

The goal of this book is to help you break this cycle by teaching you how to change the three points on the circle which keep perpetuating the problem. Turn back to the diagram of the Control Cycle and refer to it as I discuss these three skills, starting with stress and moving counter-clockwise.

Reduce stress. The first skills you will learn will be those you need to reduce stress. Since stress can impair your memory and learning abilities, it is important that this be the first skill you learn and practice. If you follow the practice guidelines diligently, you should begin to feel less stress in your daily routine in no more than a week or two. Should you still have difficulty after this period of time, you may want to supplement your new skills with autogenics training or biofeedback. Since these skills are more involved than those that you will be learning in this book, it is advisable you use them only if the relaxation techniques in this book are not working well enough. Autogenics is more complex because it is a much slower process and will take ten times longer to get the same general effect; biofeedback requires the use of equipment that can make relaxation a cumbersome process. Ideally, it is best if you need nothing more than your own mind to gain the benefits from stress reduction training. But it is important that you not be ashamed of turning to other methods should those in the following chapters prove insufficient to significantly reduce your stress.

Cognitive change. The next set of skills come from the new field in psychology called "cognitive therapy." These skills are designed to change the way you think. As you can see from the Control Cycle, your thoughts have tremendous influence over the rest of your life. In fact, they act as a bridge between what is outside of you and what happens inside of you. We all know intuitively that we are what we think, and yet we have never been shown how to change the way we think when it becomes destructive. How many times have you been told to "change your attitude" and felt helpless even though you knew it was a good idea? Mankind has been trying to change attitudes for thousands of years, but it was not until the 1970s that we began to develop the tools to do exactly that. For the first time in the history of the human race we now have the rudimentary tools for making dramatic changes in our lives by learning how to stop our negative and destructive thinking processes. As you will see when you have completed this book, this approach to the Deadly Diet is almost exclusively devoted to changing your thinking. When you change your thinking, your old habitual eating patterns won't change instantly. But they *will change*. Those thoughts, which filter out what goes on around you and which interpret your experiences, have a direct bearing on your eating behavior.

Behavior change. The last skill you will learn is the one you and everyone around you are the most concerned about. Your eating behavior is public and highly visible. Consequently, most people around you see your behavior as "the problem." How many times have others told you to "just eat more" or "stop that stupid binging and barfing." Yet you know that the eating is not the real problem. Attempts to change that focus only on the behavior are doomed because the other components of the Control Cycle have not been dealt with. To change your behavior without changing your thoughts or stress level would be like trying to put out a fire by throwing gasoline on it. It only gets worse!

The skill of behavior change is also the most scary one because it is the final step in which you have to put all your other skills into practice. It is like moving from the practice session to the stage in front of a real audience. Many people balk at this point because of what we call the plateau effect. By the time you have reached the portion of the book dealing with your actual behavior, much of your emotional pain will have been modified so that your daily life will have reached a plateau of relative comfort. Pain is a wonderful motivator, and without it many people find it difficult to make changes. When you have learned to change your destructive thoughts, it will be tempting to "take a break" from reaching your goal and to subtly and gradually begin to stop working on the problem. Beware! The plateau is not flat, but slopes backward. If you stop work at this point, you are almost assured of having a major setback that will discourage you from continuing your progress.

Three Myths

People on the Deadly Diet generally go through life believing three myths about themselves. These myths are quite powerful and can affect the way you live, your lifestyle, and your relationship to others.

MYTH 1: "I'm the only person in the world with this problem."

Some Deadly Dieters may actually not know at least one other person with the same problem. But with the current media attention focused on this problem, it is difficult to imagine that a person could believe this myth. One reason this myth is still powerful is the high denial factor that exists with Deadly Dieters. It is very common for clients to deny vehemently that they have anorexia or bulimia, while everyone around them can plainly see the problem. Although they deny the presence of the Deadly Diet, they still insist that no one else has a problem like they have, and that consequently no one can really understand or sympathize with them. If finally forced to admit that they are a Deadly Dieter, they will retreat to the conviction that "My problem is unique and totally different from the type of Deadly Diet anyone else has."

The other factor that contributes to this myth is that people don't talk about this problem in public. In many cases, it is now socially acceptable to talk about quite personal and intimate details of our lives. Few people are shocked to hear someone talking about a sexual problem, an intimate detail of their marriage, or surgery they have had. Yet it would be inappropriate for someone at a party to volunteer information about his or her Deadly Diet. This topic is rarely discussed because only another Deadly Dieter really understands it. This lack of understanding in the general population makes the Deadly Diet a very isolating problem. The person on the Deadly Diet usually begins to draw further and further away from social contact, which in turn further reinforces the myth that he or she is the only one with the problem.

MYTH 2: "My problem is incurable."

The word "incurable" is the wrong word here. The Deadly Diet has no "cure" because it is not really a medical problem. Since it is not biological in nature, there is no germ, virus, or bacteria that can be cured. The Deadly Diet can have medical side effects, but the basic problem is a learned condition, a psychological condition. The Deadly Dieter can recover by learning to conquer the problem. In this sense, being on the Deadly Diet is similar to having a problem with alcohol. It's an addiction and a handicap that may last a lifetime. But the important thing to remember is this: The solution isn't to "cure" the person, but rather to learn how to cope with the problem. Our work at the clinic has shown beyond a doubt that Deadly Diets can be brought under control.

MYTH 3: "I must be crazy or soon will be."

Once a person is absolutely convinced that she is the only person in the world with this problem and that this problem is untreatable and incurable, this third myth is unavoidable. It is very common for Deadly Dieters to believe that something is drastically wrong with them emotionally. Sometimes they are afraid that if people knew of their problem they would be sent away to a psychiatric hospital. The irony here is that people on the Deadly Diet are not only quite sane, but also generally have qualities that are admired, adored, and coveted by others. They tend to be energetic, bright, intelligent, and imaginative. Many are talented in the arts. Many of the young women with Deadly Diets are excellent students.

If you are a Deadly Dieter, it's very important to know that you are not going to go crazy! You may feel like you are losing your grasp on reality, especially if other people don't understand the problem. But remember—you are a normal person with a very difficult problem.

2

Stress

A cold shudder shakes my limbs, and my chilled blood freezes with terror.

—VERGIL, 19 B.C.

Stress is a problem that many people misunderstand. One reason is that stress is often confused with its causes or seen as being equivalent to the pressures that trigger it—all the demands, all the uncertainties, all the "stresses." Some people have become quite sophisticated in understanding stress triggers. For example, participants in stress reduction programs spend a considerable amount of time learning how to compute their "change life units," how to manage their time, how to minimize daily pressures, and how to deal more assertively with demands from others. Other stress triggers that people learn how to cope with are having a deadline that can't be met, not having enough money to pay bills, dealing with death or separation, or having someone pressure you to change a behavior. But to understand what stress is really all about, you must know that all these "stresses" merely serve to bring stress on. These triggers are not stress itself.

Another form of misunderstanding confuses stress with what it does to our bodies and our emotional well-being. Medicine has finally admitted that many illnesses and diseases can be brought on or made worse by stress. For example, stress is clearly a factor in heart disease. Hypertension has also been linked with our immunological system and its ability to fight disease. Typical signs of stress are headache, insomnia, change of appetite, dizziness, fatigue, nausea, and irritability. Yet you must realize that all of these physical complaints are merely symptoms of stress. They also are not stress itself.

What Is Stress?

Although our society has become quite familiar with the triggers and symptoms of stress, we still don't have a good understanding of what stress really is. When a weekly news magazine recently featured a cover story on stress, one of the nation's leading experts was quoted as saying that he did not know exactly what stress was. At the California Clinic, we have developed our own working definition. Stress is not an emotion or an abstract idea, nor is it something that is difficult to understand. It is an event—a concrete and tangible event. This event is composed of three basic biological components. Stress is simply the combination of:

1. Improper breathing
2. Body/muscle tension
3. A racing mind

These three things do not cause stress. Nor are they the result of stress. Rather THEY ARE STRESS. Think about it—when you are stressed, your breathing is rapid and shallow, your muscles become tense, and your mind races so fast that it seems to be going in fifty different directions at the same time. Now look at these components from another point of view. Imagine yourself breathing very gently, slowly, and naturally; imagine yourself having released all muscle tension from your body; imagine calming your mind down. What would you feel like? When I ask my clients this question, the reply is usually a one-word answer: "Wonderful!"

Stress Triggers	Stress	Stress Effects
Tests in school	Insomnia	Improper breathing
Fight with friend	Muscle tension	Hypertension
Too many things to do	Mind racing	Headaches
New job demands		Fatigue
Death of a loved one		Poor memory

Stress is not something that is simply turned on or off. Although excessive stress is the opposite of relaxation, there is a large middle ground consisting of varying degrees of stress. Some people find it helpful to think of stress existing on a ten-point scale. Very few of us would experience a zero or a ten very often in our lives. Most of us would find that, on the average, our stress levels would vary between four and six. Maybe it would go up to a seven or even an eight on a particularly hectic day. And maybe it would drop to a two or three on an especially relaxing day. During a typical day we may have to breathe rapidly at times, we may have to tense our muscles, we may have to make our mind move quickly.

So far I have been using the word "stress" as if it were a thing to be avoided. In fact, we are all "stressed" just by being alive. By going about our daily business we have to stress ourselves—by breathing rapidly, tensing our muscles, and speeding up our thoughts. When we talk about stress as a problem, we are really talking about the excessive accumulation of stress. This over-accumulation of stress may result from overreacting to a given situation by breathing too quickly when it is unnecessary, tensing too much when it serves no purpose, or letting your mind race when there is no reason for it to do so.

Methods of Stress Reduction

There are really two ways of dealing with stress: a prevention method and a crisis method. These two methods of stress reduction are similar to two methods commonly used to solve other types of problems.

Close to where I live are the foothills that begin the Sierra Nevadas. Because of the state's need to provide water to its ever-increasing population, California has built many reservoirs in these hills. Sometimes, when we have had a particularly wet winter, the melting of the snowpack in the spring can threaten an overflow of the reservoirs. Those responsible for this condition theoretically have two methods available to them for keeping the danger of a flood at a minimum: prevention and crisis. Both of these solutions are legitimate, yet the two are very different ways of attacking the problem.

The crisis method would avert flood problems by responding directly to the amount of water behind the dam. The engineers in charge would simply open the dam and let the water flow out of the reservoir faster than it came in. Similarly, the crisis method for dealing with stress is to get the stress out of your body as quickly as possible—faster than it is coming in. By learning how to use this method effectively and quickly, you can let yourself stay in the high stress situation and yet feel relaxed, calm, and unstressed.

In theory, the second method—the prevention method—would simply stop the snow from melting. Although this may seem like an impractical way of coping with mountain snows and reservoirs, the idea does work when we are dealing with stress reduction. Remember that stress is internally generated. It occurs because of what you think. If you can learn to change your thoughts, then you can learn how to prevent stress from becoming excessive.

The combination of these two methods will provide you with two tools for dealing with stress. The prevention method will keep you from becoming unduly stressed, which means that your life in general will become more relaxed and calm. Should you find yourself in a situation where the stress is building too rapidly, you will then have the crisis method to relieve yourself of the excessive stress. In this chapter you will learn how to use the crisis method; in later chapters you will learn how to use the "prevention method" of stress control.

Techniques of Stress Reduction

Since stress is a combination of improper breathing, tense muscles, and a racing mind, you will need to learn three skills to counteract each of these three stress components. To control your breathing, you will learn a system I call *Natural Breathing*. There are many different ways of getting your muscles relaxed, but the one that seems to work the best for most people is a technique called *Progressive Relaxation. Mental Imagery* can be used to calm your mind. Although this technique is often used in a somewhat mystical fashion, it is really a very straightforward way of obtaining peace of mind. Although these three skills can be learned by anyone, you will still need to put considerable time and effort into learning them and mastering them. You must also remember that the three skills are not of equal difficulty. While you can learn and master Natural Breathing in a matter of days and Progressive Relaxation in a matter of weeks, calming your mind will probably take you months of effort. Don't let these varying degrees of difficulty discourage you. Several months from now, when you are doing well with other skills but the Mental Imagery is still hard, just remember this is normally the most difficult of the stress reduction skills.

Natural Breathing

This is an effective, quick technique that can be used literally anywhere and any time. If you have ever hyperventilated, Natural Breathing will keep you from ever doing this again for the rest of your life. This is because hyperventilation and Natural Breathing are incompatible—they cannot happen at the same time. You cannot sit and stand at the same time because they, too, are incompatible. When you master Natural Breathing, you won't ever have to carry a paper bag with you again! Natural Breathing has three components: deep breathing, slow breathing, and discontinuous breathing.

Deep breathing. To learn to breathe deeply, you first need to check how you currently take a deep breath. Do this now by standing in front of a mirror. As you take a really deep breath, watch what happens to your upper body and your stomach. You may notice that your upper body will move—if you took a really big breath, you may have raised your shoulders—and your stomach will be drawn in. Although the vast majority of the human race takes a deep breath in this way, it is wrong. It is wrong because it is backwards.

For a truly deep breath to occur, there must be little or no movement in your upper body—and at the same time your stomach must be pushed out. (This "belly breathing" is used by professional musicians.) To learn how to breathe deeply properly, put your hands on your stomach, directly on top of your navel. Now push in. While you are pushing in, push your hands away from your body with your stomach muscles. Then, as you relax your stomach muscles, let your hands push your stomach back in again. This in-and-out movement of your stomach muscles is the same movement that should occur when you breathe deeply.

Now that you have experienced this movement in your stomach muscles, you know which muscles to use for deep breathing. To learn the complete technique of natural deep breathing, follow this simple four-step procedure. (This procedure should always be done by inhaling and exhaling through your mouth.) (1) Push your stomach in again with your hands. (2) Let the air out of your lungs (be sure to keep your stomach pushed in). (3) Now "breathe in, push out" and (4) "breathe out push in." When you do this for the first time, it should feel different from any other kind of breathing you have experienced before. It may feel either labored or easy depending on how quickly you can adjust to the new coordination of your stomach muscles with your breathing patterns.

Do this several more times so that you can get the feel of what is happening to you. Don't despair if it doesn't come easy. If you are a woman, you have two strikes against you in learning this procedure. First, you must counteract years of physical conditioning. You have been breathing incorrectly for many years, and it may take some time for you to coordinate your muscles. Second, social conditioning has taught you that, as a woman, "you must never push your stomach out." Let me reassure you that the first problem will take care of itself very quickly. The second is really nonexistent. When you learn to do this naturally, you can deep breathe and nobody will notice it.

Breathing slowly. Now that you have learned to breathe deeply, you must also learn how to breathe more slowly. If you breathe *quickly* and deeply, you will not get the full benefit of Natural Breathing. You can learn to breathe slowly by simply spelling the word "relax" to yourself as you breathe in and again as you breathe out. Spell the word silently at the rate of about one letter per second. In this way it will take you about five to six seconds to inhale and the same amount of time to exhale. A total breathe cycle will last about ten to twelve seconds (which means about five or six breaths a minute). This will probably feel a lot slower than the breathing you are used to. Try this now (using the four-part procedure for deep breathing you just learned) and see how slowly you can breathe. It would be unusual for you to get past the "L" in relax," because most people take in a quick breath and then try to slow it down for the remaining four seconds.

Musicians know that the secret to slow breathing is something called "breath control." When you begin to inhale, do it very gently and gradually, moving your stomach very slowly. You will probably find that controlling the speed of exhaling will be easier than controlling the speed of inhaling.

Breathing discontinuously. Finally, you need to learn how to breathe discontinuously. Listen to your breathing for a few seconds as you normally do it. You will notice that your exhaling and inhaling flow from one to the other. To breathe naturally, you must learn to pause after you exhale and before you take in another breath. How long this pause takes is insignificant. The important factor is that you put a discrete, specific pause between the exhale and the inhale. This pause will help you to further slow down your breathing. Remember, the pause is the opposite of holding your breath. When you hold your breath, you stop breathing while your lungs are full of air; when you pause, you stop breathing when your lungs empty.

I have named this type of breathing "Natural Breathing" for a good reason: this is the way you naturally breathed when you were born. If you watch a baby on its back, you will notice the little tummy going slowly up and down as it breathes. When the stomach comes down on the exhale, there is a long pause before another breath is taken. So, you see, you are not learning anything new. Rather, you are relearning how to do something that your body considers natural and that which you have been *taught* not to do.

Now that you know how to breathe naturally, it is imperative that you also learn how to do it automatically. When you are stressed, it can be extremely difficult to remember a half-learned skill. To make Natural Breathing a regular part of your life, you need to practice this skill on a consistent basis. Instructions for practicing your Natural Breathing will be found at the end of this chapter.

Progressive Relaxation

There are many ways to release muscle tension, all of which can work quite well. If you already have a favorite method and it is currently working for you, you may want to continue using it. But for beginners, the method used in this book is probably the easiest of all available methods: (1) the muscle feedback you receive while you are using this method helps you to quickly identify what relaxation feels like; (2) it relies on no external devices (biofeedback instruments) to tell you when you are relaxed; and (3) it is capable of being streamlined so that its inherent clumsiness is eventually eliminated.

Streamlining your relaxation. Let's explore this last feature more thoroughly. Progressive Relaxation, which was discovered in the 1930s, is very powerful and effective, but at the same time very inconvenient and awkward. First, it usually takes about twenty minutes of your time when you first learn the skill. And to learn it well you need to practice it several times a day. Unfortunately, in our busy world very few people have the necessary time, no matter how motivated and well-meaning they are. But as you perfect this skill, you will be shown how to speed up the process. Eventually, should you choose to put in the work, you can learn how to relax in less than thirty seconds.

Second, you will be learning to use Progressive Relaxation with your eyes closed. This helps to minimize the distractions that hinder the learning of any new skill. However, if you can only relax when your eyes are closed, you are somewhat limited as to when and where you can relax. You will also be shown how to relax with your eyes open in later chapters.

Third, you need to minimize auditory distractions at first so that you can better concentrate on what you are learning. This is somewhat irrelevant to the real world, because not many people need to relax when it is quiet and calm. So, you will also be shown how to relax in a noisy environment.

Fourth, you will initially relax in a comfortable sitting position. But, again, very few people have nice comfortable chairs scattered around their world to sit down in when the need for relaxation arises. You will also be taught how to relax standing up and walking around.

Finally, you must learn how to be inconspicuous when you relax. If the only way you can relax is by tensing and releasing your muscles, you are somewhat limited as to where this can be done. You will also need to relax just as deeply without first tensing your muscles.

It is also important that you understand how to streamline this relaxation exercise, because you may be reluctant to practice several times a day when you find out how inconvenient it is. By realizing that the relaxation can become more efficient, you will have more incentive to continue a skill that can only help to improve the quality of your life.

There are two ways of learning Progressive Relaxation. You can either have a friend read the instructions for you the first time, or you can record the instructions yourself on tape. The first time you try Progressive Relaxation, you can listen to the tape and follow the instructions. But after this first time, I want you to practice your progressive relaxation WITHOUT listening to the tape. Although you will find it more difficult to relax without listening to the tape, it will work better for you in the long run. It is too easy to get hooked on the tape for relaxation—it becomes a mechanical Valium. I want the tape inside your head, not inside a tape recorder.

Either way you choose, make sure the instructions are read slowly, in a fairly monotonous but clear voice. You need to be in a room with as few distractions as possible (or you can be outside if this works best for you). Be sure that the television and radio are off, the telephone is unplugged, and all pets are in another room or outside. Although many people think that relaxation is done best lying down, I have found this hinders you in the long run. When you are starting out, always practice your Progressive Relaxation sitting up. Preferably you want a high-backed chair or some other type of arrangement that can support your head.

You will notice that the muscle relaxation instructions are immediately followed by a set of simple instructions for calming your mind down. Do not be concerned if you find your mind wandering. It will take months of practice before you can correct this natural tendency.

Use the following instructions word for word unless you have a compelling reason for changing them. These words and phrases have been revised countless numbers of times to help you obtain the best relaxation possible. When you see a series of dots within the instructions (. . . .), each dot stands for a one-second pause. You should read these instructions slowly. They should take about fifteen to twenty minutes to complete.

Progressive Relaxation/Mental Imagery

You're going to go through an exercise that many people in our speeded up and tense society could profit from doing on a regular basis. This exercise is basically simple, and in its simplicity lies its importance. One might say you knew more about relaxing as an infant than you do as an adult. This ability to relax like an infant is what you can achieve through practicing this exercise. I want you to experience, now, for a brief period, that blissful, carefree relaxation of infancy. But first, to realize the experience of relaxation, it is important for you to feel the full effect of its opposite, namely tension, throughout your body. To do this I would like you to focus your complete attention on each part of your body as I mention it.

TAPE

First, concentrate all of your attention on your RIGHT FOOT and the toes of this foot. With your right foot flat on the floor, lift your toes upward and fan them outward. This will create tension in your ankle and the calf of your right leg. . . . Now relax it quickly, just let go completely. . . .

Next, focus on your LEFT FOOT and toes. Extend your left toes upward and fan them out as far as they will go. Once again there will be a feeling of tension in your ankle and calf. . . . Now, relax your left foot completely. When I ask you to release the tension, try to let go as much as possible. The secret in relaxing is in the letting go.

Now tense the muscles in your RIGHT THIGH by pressing down with your right heel. Press down really hard on the heel of your right foot . . . feel the tension. . . . Now relax your heel and thigh—let go and notice the difference. In fact, each time you let go try to identify the difference in feeling between tension and relaxation. Notice how pleasant it feels just to have your muscles relaxing and letting go.

Let's do the same thing with your LEFT THIGH. Tense it as tightly as you can by pressing down with your left heel. Press down hard with your left heel and feel the tension as much as possible. . . . Let go and relax all over. . . . You may have noticed by now a pleasant sensation arising as you relax a group of muscles.

Next, focus on your STOMACH muscles, your abdomen. Tighten your stomach muscles into a hard knot. Keep your stomach as hard as you can for just a little while and notice that tension. . . . Now relax, just let go, let all your body muscles loosen completely, and notice the difference once again. . . . You may notice an inner feeling of well-being coming over you as you are able to relax more and more of your muscles. But you need to remember that relaxing is not something that you do, but something you allow to happen. You cannot force it, because it is a perfectly natural response to letting go. You were born knowing how to relax. All you need to do now is to allow it to happen. Just let go.

Next, direct your attention to your LOWER BACK—arch up your back. Arch your back way up and make your back taut and hollow and feel the tension up and down your spine. . . . Now, relax and sit back comfortably again. As you let go, try to remember that there is no limit to the amount of relaxation you can personally experience. Theoretically, you can relax to the point of infinity. Go ahead and relax your back—relax your body as much as possible. . . . Just relax further and further, letting the relaxation go deeper and deeper into your muscles.

While you keep the rest of your body relaxed, I want you to clench your RIGHT FIST. Clench your fist tighter and tighter . . . study the tension in your hand and arm as you do this. . . . Now relax and let the fingers of your hand become loose, completely loose. Notice how different your arm and your hand feel.

Next, clench your LEFT FIST, really tight. Clench it really tight and notice the tension in that arm. . . . Now, let go. Relax your left fingers. Let them straighten out and become limp. . . . Notice the difference once again.

Next, bend your RIGHT ELBOW and bring the fingers of your right hand up to your right shoulder. With your fingers touching your shoulder, tense the muscles of your right arm hard. . . . Study that tension in your bicep. . . . All right, straighten out your arm and let go. . . . Just relax all your muscles and feel the warm, pleasant heaviness that comes with relaxing completely.

Let's do the same thing with your LEFT ARM. Touch your shoulder and tense your left bicep tightly. . . . Hold that tension really tightly and observe it carefully. . . . Let go, let out your left arm. Let it, too, drop limp—relax it as much as you can. . . . Try to let yourself actually feel the relaxation. Continue to let go. Let your whole body relax further and further into deeper and still deeper levels of relaxation.

Now, let's focus on your NECK muscles. Press your head back as far as you can. Press it back hard, really hard. . . . Feel the tension in your neck. Hold that tension briefly. . . . Let go. Let your neck relax as much as possible. Let the muscles loosen so completely that your head is as heavy as a bowling ball. Allow the back of the chair to completely support your head so that your neck muscles can relax totally and completely.

Next, hunch up both of your SHOULDERS. Bring your shoulders right up to your ears. Feel the tension. . . . Now drop your shoulders, let them go completely limp and feel the relaxation. . . . Let that relaxation go deeper and deeper into your shoulders—then let it filter right down into the rest of your body.

Now, raise your eyebrows so that it makes your FOREHEAD and the top of your SCALP all tight and wrinkly. . . . Feel the tension. . . . Relax your forehead, smooth it out. Try to picture, as in a mirror, your forehead becoming smoother and smoother as the relaxation increases.

Next, squeeze your EYES tightly shut . . . tighter and tighter. Feel the tension in your eyelids. . . . Relax them and keep your eyes closed gently and comfortably. Notice how relaxed they feel.

Finally, let's tense the muscles around your MOUTH. Clench your jaws and lips. Clench them tightly together and study the tension around your mouth. . . . Relax those muscles, let your cheeks and lips hang loose, limp. Relax your jaw and keep your teeth slightly apart as you continue to relax all the muscles around your mouth.

Try to notice the contrast throughout your entire body between tension and relaxation. If any tension has crept back into your body, release it and let it go. . . . In your mind's eye, picture your face as though looking in a mirror and actually see the relaxation all over your face. Observe the relaxation around your mouth . . . notice it around your eyes . . . see it all over your forehead. . . . Actually feel the relaxation progress further and further. Just allow yourself to feel the relaxation take over and go deeper and deeper, and still deeper into the muscles and very fiber of your body.

As you become more and more deeply relaxed, your body may feel very heavy. It is also possible that parts of your body may feel very small or maybe even quite large. You may also feel warm all over, or perhaps parts of your body have no feeling—for instance, maybe a hand or foot even feels like it is disconnected from the rest of your body. Whatever you feel as you sit there completely relaxed, just go along with it and enjoy it. Let it happen without bothering to control or question it. The reason is that these things are perfectly natural in a deeply relaxed state. They are normal, for instance, when you are drifting off to sleep; but the difference here is that you can let your mind go blank or let your thoughts drift around without going to sleep. Let yourself feel calm and peaceful . . . warm and relaxed.

The final part of training in relaxation is the most important part, because it is concerned with mentally letting go as well as physically relaxing, of getting rid of cares and frustrations and mentally relaxing without going to sleep. To begin, I want you to picture in your mind's eye a scene representing pure, unconditional pleasure to you. Just give yourself the mental set to picture what you're thinking as you sit there, completely relaxed with your eyes closed.

You may want to concentrate on something you have experienced recently, or perhaps you remember something wonderful about a vacation you've taken, or you may recall something you've seen in a movie or read in a book. It is even possible to think of some happy event that may have occurred while you were in the middle of some hectic activity. Of course, you may want to recall something serene or pleasurable from your childhood.

Whatever comes to you, let it be your private experience to feel fully again for just a little while. Let your mind drift peacefully and relaxed wherever it wants to go. If your mind begins to wander, don't be concerned or fight it. Rather, gently bring your mind back to the scene you have chosen. I am going to remain silent for a few moments while you allow yourself to follow anything pleasant . . . happy . . . or peaceful that appears to you. Let it take you wherever you want to go, just drifting and enjoying. After a few moments of silence I am going to count forward from one to five while you then bring yourself back to the present, at which time you will arouse yourself, refreshed and calm.

* * * TWO-MINUTE PAUSE * * *

Please keep your eyes closed until you are asked to open them. It is now time to come back to the present. But you may have been relaxed for so long in this session that it may take a minute or two for you to become fully alert again. This is to be expected at first, but with regular practice you will find that you can become relaxed very quickly, and that when you have refreshed yourself in this way you will always be able to arouse yourself effectively by counting from ~~one~~ to ~~five~~. This counting will always bring you back from your deep relaxation fully alert and refreshed with all physical exertion and emotional strain gone.

I'll count for you this time. You may wish to count silently to yourself along with me.

5 ~~One.~~ You are more aware of the present and finding yourself more refreshed and more invigorated than you have ever been in your whole life.

4 ~~Two.~~ It's time to stir about by moving your feet and legs. Remember, when you open your eyes, you will be refreshed as though you were awakening from a long nap.

3 ~~Three.~~ You might want to stretch your arms out. From head to foot you are feeling perfect: mentally, physically, and emotionally.

2 ~~Four.~~ Now you should move your head around a bit. You are now completely refreshed, rejuvenated, and ready to open your eyes.

1 ~~Five.~~ Open your eyes!

Panic Attacks

(If you are a Deadly Dieter who does not experience panic attacks, feel free to skip this section.)

Some Deadly Dieters accumulate so much stress that they experience panic attacks. It must be remembered that a panic attack is really nothing more than a physical reaction. It occurs when too much adrenalin shoots into your bloodstream too quickly. Anyone can experience a panic attack by having adrenalin injected into their veins.

A panic attack is difficult to describe to an individual who has never had one. For those who have them, it is a *terrifying* experience. Some of the physical symptoms accompanying attacks are heart palpitations, weakness and exhaustion, dizziness, "jelly knees," missed heartbeats, inability to take a deep breath, blurred vision, aching muscles, an illusion of walking on shifting ground, a sense of isolation and unreality, and an urge to escape and find safety.

A panic attack is different from an anxiety attack. An anxiety attack is an excess of anxiety. A panic attack is an excess of stress. It is a necessary mechanism built into our genetic makeup that keeps us alive. We know that excessive stress in metals can cause them to break and be destroyed. The same thing applies to the human body: excessive stress can literally destroy the body. Panic attacks are the body's way of caring for itself by stopping the individual from building up any more stress when the limit has been reached. The panic attack causes a person to immediately stop what he or she is doing and to do something to relieve the excess stress.

Coping With Panic Attacks

For those of you who have panic attacks, you will be able to deal successfully with them by the time you have finished this book. Until then, you can follow seven simple steps for handling a panic attack.

STEP 1. _Don 't fight the panic_. Let it come! When you feel the panic mount, let the feelings come. They cannot hurt you. Try to "float" your way through the panic. What does it mean to "float" through a panic attack? Have you ever gone swimming in the ocean, and noticed how hard it was to fight the waves and resist the strong tidal surge? Even the most powerful and skilled swimmers are no match for mother nature and the Pacific Ocean.

When a smart swimmer gets caught in a rough predicament, she doesn't fight the current. Instead, she RELAXES her body, bobs like a cork, and FLOATS with the ocean swells. So it is with the panic. When you feel panicky, visualize your feelings as a passing ocean swell. Remember the swimmer: she floats, she does not fight. She relaxes, she does not tense. She accepts, she does not panic.

The more you do this, the more control you will have, and the sooner the panic will evaporate. Remember, when the panic begins to mount, let the feelings come, accept them, float with them, and let your body go limp. Let the oncoming tide of panic rise and fall—and it will fall if you let it.

STEP 2. _Engage in repetitive, constructive, positive thinking._ For years, you've been pumping up your fears and fueling your panic fires with words like: "OH NO! Here comes those awful feelings. I can't stand it! I'm trapped—out of control!" Sound familiar? And sure enough, you felt afraid, trapped, and out of control, NOT BECAUSE OF THE SITUATION, BUT BECAUSE OF THE WORDS YOU WERE TELLING YOURSELF.

Change your vocabulary and say goodbye to panic. Instead of using words that exaggerate and distort, begin to engage in rational, constructive, and positive thinking when you feel a panic attack coming on. If you "de-awfulize" episodes of severe stress, then the panic subsides, and the panic monster is beheaded. Believe me, it works. You _can_ do it! These are not just empty words of encouragement—they are words of truth. Just believing in your own power over panic is your most powerful weapon in overcoming panic.

STEP 3. _Start your Natural Breathing, Muscle Relaxation, and Mental Imagery_. Three things happen when you panic: (l) your body tenses, (2) your mind begins to race, and (3) your breathing is quick and shallow.

So in panic situations, it is very important to begin to take deep, SLOOOOW, discontinuous breaths from the stomach. Other people will not notice that you are breathing deeply and from the stomach. Remember to tense and release various muscles in your body. And finally, try to think of a pleasant, relaxing scene as vividly as possible.

Now, of course, everyone knows that these things are next to impossible to do when you are caught in the undertow of a panic attack. Nevertheless, *any* attempt to use these skills is better than nothing at all.

STEP 4. *Wait for the panic to subside.* Get as comfortable as possible, but do not run. Stay put. Then float, breathe, accept, think constructively, and the panic will subside. It must! Your body cannot maintain a panic reaction for very long if you float with it and let go. By tensing and resisting it you are adding fuel to the fire and keeping the panic attack going. So, let go. That's the key—letting go, as if you were floating in space.

STEP 5. *After it's over, look on the episode as a success.* After all, you made it! It was either a positive time (you used these suggestions and faced the panic), or else it was a learning time (what would you do differently next time?). Release guilty self-talk like "I really blew it, I shouldn't have panicked," and so on. In so far as your feelings are concerned, there is no right and wrong, no good and bad. Guilt will slow or halt your progress.

STEP 6. *Look forward to your next panic attack.* With that attitude, the panic will begin to disappear by itself.

STEP 7. *Don't worry about your racing heart, tight stomach, feelings of unreality and isolation.* They are just symptoms of panicky stress— period! They go away when the panic fades.

Panic Episodes as Learning Opportunities

Begin to view panic attacks as a time to practice and recover. Admittedly, panic attacks are uncomfortable, inconvenient, and not much fun. But the sooner you begin to face your panic, float through it, and count your successes, the sooner the panic attacks will go away.

Opportunity is knocking. Letting go of panic is a learned skill. With time and practice, you will soon gain the upper hand over panic, like thousands of others just like you.

Give yourself time. Remember that you don't have to handle your next panic attack perfectly. Success does not mean going from failure to perfection the first time out. Relief comes by using these tools again and again until you gain control over your stress.

Each time you make it through a panic attack, put an entry into your success log or journal. "I made it! I'm still breathing, still alive, and unharmed! I'm taking charge of my stress and panic!"

Assessing Body Tension

Earlier, I suggested you think of stress as existing on a ten-point scale. This idea will help you to more accurately measure your own body tension. On this scale, a one represents minimum stress and a ten stands for the maximum stress—a panic attack. Unfortunately, many people don't realize they are stressed until they have reached the upper levels like seven or eight. If you can learn to recognize stress around three and four, you will find it much easier to keep your stress level from escalating out of control.

John Travis, in his *Wellness Workbook*, has developed a series of exercises* designed to help you discover how much body tension you actually have. By using these exercises, you can begin to recognize your stress levels and catch the stress at an earlier stage.

Bracing

Chronic bracing or tensing of your muscles may go completely unnoticed, yet leave you drained of energy at the end of the day. It may also lead to many muscular disorders. "Bracing" is something like sitting in your car at a traffic light with one foot pressed down on the accelerator and the other foot on the brake. There is no movement, but much energy is expended with extra wear on the engine, transmission, and brakes. The same is true of a body that is continually braced, whether you notice it or not.

> *Exercise 1.* With your knees locked, bend over without straining and try to touch your fingers to your toes. Record the number of inches that you are short of touching your toes ("-2"), or if you can just touch them, record a "0." If you can easily reach further, estimate how many inches beyond your toes you can reach. For instance, palms flat on the floor might be "+ 6," depending on the size of your hands.

This exercise will provide you with a general measure of your flexibility. Bracing leads to a lack of flexibility—often erroneously attributed to aging. If your body is in good shape and you are not doing a lot of bracing, your flexibility should be "+" several inches, even if you are past middle age.

---

*Reprinted with permission, *Wellness Workbook*, Copyright 1977, 1981, John W. Travis, M.D., Ryan and Travis, Ten Speed Press, Berkeley, CA.

Wrinkle Patterns

Until you are about thirty years old, the natural elasticity of your skin will resist permanent wrinkling from muscle tension, although exposure to excessive sunlight and cigarette smoke will break down the elastic fibers sooner. After thirty, muscles that are tensed will begin to etch permanent lines into your face. Expressions characteristic of chronic emotional stress will often appear. For example, persons who are frequently angry, yet rarely experience or express anger, may take on a permanent scowl and a furrowed brow. Others may have sad, fearful, or puzzled looks.

> *Exercise 2.* Look in a mirror. Notice any wrinkles in your forehead or around your eyes or mouth.
>
> Do you find any signs or patterns of muscle tension in your face?
>
> Look at any lines you have and exaggerate them by tightening the muscles which formed the lines. Notice any emotions you experience while tightening the muscles.
>
> Are your legs, thighs, shoulders, or other parts of your body often tense?

Symptoms or diseases which often go with excessive muscle tension are: backaches, neck and back problems, baldness, arthritis, asthma, high blood pressure, stroke, and heart disease.

Heart Rate

Rapid pulse rates result from lack of exercise, from chronic anxiety, and from chemicals like nicotine or caffeine. All of these things can be quite stressful to your body.

> *Exercise 3.* Find your pulse, either in your neck on either side of your Adam's apple or in your wrist. While sitting or lying in a relaxed position, count your pulse for one full minute.
>
> Do you smoke or drink coffee? If so, go without them a few days and notice any change in your pulse rate.

Circulation to Hands and Feet

Another way the body manifests stress is by cutting off blood flow to the hands and feet. In an emergency, this process is designed to allow more blood to go to the muscles where it is needed most. When blood flow to the extremities is reduced, the result is cold hands and feet—a common complaint among Deadly Dieters.

Exercise 4. Make sure that you are in an environment of about 70°F. Take your hand temperature with a thermometer. You can do this by grasping the bulb of a thermometer between your index finger and thumb. Allow about one minute for the temperature to stabilize—then read the thermometer.

If the thermometer reads under 85° F, you are probably constricting blood flow to your hands. This indicates unnecessary body tension. You may want to carry the thermometer with you and record your hand temperature several times a day, especially at times when you suspect you might be stressed.

By relaxing and focusing on warming your hands, you can raise your hand temperature as much as 20 degrees in five minutes. The result of warming your hands to 95 or 96° F is usually a deep state of relaxation. You may want to check this by taking your hand temperature immediately after doing your Progressive Relaxation exercise.

Perspiration

Sweat gland activity is another window into a body's inner storehouse of tension. The sympathetic nervous system controls many activities in your skin, the most noticeable of which is sweat production. Chronic tension can lead to chronic moistness of the hands, feet, brow, or armpits.

Exercise 5. Notice if your hands, feet, armpits, brow, or other parts are moist now. If not, recall times when you experienced this moistness. Is it frequent? Can you correlate that moistness with any emotions or stressful situations?

Homework

Now that you know how to eliminate stress from your body, it is important that you master the skills involved by practicing them on a regular basis. The following schedule will help you to become proficient.

/· Natural Breathing

Begin right now by taking five Natural Breaths (deeply, slowly, discontinuously). An hour from now do the same thing. Continue taking five Natural Breaths per hour for the next day or two. If you will stick to this schedule conscientiously, you should be able to master Natural Breathing within twenty four to forty eight hours. Eventually, you will be able to breathe naturally by merely thinking of it—any time, any where.

When you first begin practicing Natural Breathing, you may notice that you get light-headed. If this happens, it means that you are breathing improperly, probably too shallowly. But if you ever feel like yawning when doing your breathing exercises, this means that you are breathing absolutely correctly—because a yawn is an exaggerated Natural Breath. When you yawn, you yawn deeply and slowly and pause when you are finished.

There are three stages to mastering Natural Breathing. The first is to practice every hour until it can be done merely by thinking of it. Second, after it can be done spontaneously, you need to practice Natural Breathing in as many settings as you possibly can. Practice it sitting, standing, and lying down; practice it while watching TV, eating, talking with friends, and even exercising. When you have learned to "generalize" this skill to a variety of situations, you are ready for the third stage. That is, you can now just do it when you need it. Nobody breathes like this all the time. But it is helpful to do it when you are feeling uptight, tense, or nervous.

2. Progressive Relaxation

To get the full benefit of muscle relaxation, you need to practice this exercise at least four times each day—preferably the first thing in the morning, around mid to late morning, mid to late afternoon, and finally early evening. A typical schedule may look like this: 7:00 A.M., 11:00 A.M., 3:00 P.M., and 7:00 P.M. These sessions are about four hours apart.

If you happen to work during these times, you can improvise and still get your practice sessions in. For example, you could practice in the morning before going to work, during your lunch hour, after you get home from work, and then in the evening. It may be that your schedule is such that it is literally impossible to practice during your lunch hour. This means you will just have to live with only three practice sessions a day.

It is best if you keep a record of your relaxation sessions. Record keeping has been found to be one of the most effective ways to improve self-discipline. You can use the chart on the next page for this purpose. This record sheet is fairly self-explanatory, except for the last column. In this column you may want to put a number from one to five, indicating how successful you thought your practice was.

3. Mental Imagery

Practicing your stress reduction four times a day can make it difficult after awhile to come up with meaningful images. If you begin to find it hard to think of pleasant things, try using these scenes to trigger your own creative imagination.

Relaxation Sessions Record				
Date	Time	Type of Relaxation	Time Spent	Rating

- Imagine that you are listening to your favorite musical selection.
- Imagine that you are playing with a friendly dog.
- Imagine the most beautiful scene you have ever experienced.
- Imagine that you are swimming in cool, clear water on a very hot day.
- Imagine that the person whom you most admire says, "WOW, you really look terrific today."
- Imagine that the person whom you most admire says, "Gee, you're pretty bright."
- Imagine that you are eating your favorite flavor of ice cream.
- Imagine that you are eating your favorite type of pastry.
- Imagine eating your favorite kind of candy.
- Imagine that you are looking at a handsome man (or beautiful woman).
- Imagine that you are lying on a beautiful, uncrowded beach.
- Imagine that you are sitting under a tree beside a beautiful, clear mountain lake.
- Imagine that you are drinking your favorite cold drink on a hot day.
- Imagine that you are eating your favorite type of food.
- Imagine the sexiest situation that you can imagine.
- Imagine that you are watching your favorite sport.
- Imagine that you are playing your favorite sport.
- Imagine that you are smelling your favorite odor (a flower, some type of food, the ocean, etc.).
- Imagine that you have just been outside on a cold, snowy day; you are now in front of a bright, warm fire and sipping hot coffee.
- Imagine that you have just finished work on Friday and are looking forward to a week of vacation.
- Imagine that you are driving (or riding) in your brand new car on a beautiful day.

- Imagine that you have just finished solving a puzzle at a party that no one else could solve.

- You are at a party and a person you think is very attractive is flirting with you.

- Imagine that you are taking a shower because you feel tired and sweaty after working hard all day.

- Imagine that you have just told a joke to a group of people and everyone is laughing a lot.

- Imagine that a doctor has just examined you thoroughly and says, "You are really in terrific shape now."

- Imagine that you have just received a telegram announcing that you have won $25,000 in a contest.

- Imagine that you are at work and your supervisor says to you, "You know, your work really has been excellent."

- Imagine that you have walked into a nudist colony by mistake and a very attractive nude person smiles and says, "Can I help you?"

- Imagine that you are in an elevator and the person riding with you is your favorite entertainer. He smiles and says, "Hi."

Morning Rituals

One of the most difficult things for the Deadly Dieter to control is time. In the next chapter I will show you a simple technique for learning to budget your time. Right now, I want you to begin bracketing your day with a set of rituals each morning and another set of rituals each evening. You will begin with one ritual in the morning and one in the evening. We will add more as we continue through the book. These rituals are meant to help you start each day off properly so that you don't just get up each morning and begin the same old Deadly Diet rat race. The evening rituals are designed to keep any problems from spilling over into the next day.

For your first morning ritual, I want you to read the following set of statements to yourself, aloud, in the mirror, at the beginning of each day. These statements are meant to help you to remember to slow down.

Slowing Down

I will slow myself down.

I will ease the pounding of my heart by the quieting of my mind.

I will steady my hurried pace with a vision of the eternal reach of time.

I will give myself, amid the confusion of the day, the calmness of the everlasting hills.

I will break the tensions of my nerves and muscles with the soothing music of the singing of streams that lives in my memory.

I will give myself the magical, restoring power of sleep.

I will take minute vacations by slowing down to look at each flower, to chat with a friend, to pat a dog, or to read a few lines from a good book.

I will be inspired to send my roots deep into the soil of life's enduring so that I may grow toward the stars of my greater destiny.

Evening Rituals

Every night, before going to bed, set aside time to identify all of the successes you have had during the day. To do this, keep a section in your notebook for a Success Journal. Write in this section all the successes you have during the day. There is a catch, however Your successes, and this is important to remember, are *only* those assignments that you have had up to this point. This is extremely critical, because you have, more than likely, always measured your success or failure against your eating behavior. You are not ready yet to deal with your eating directly, so it would be foolish to use this behavior as a standard for success.

The definition of success is limited to only those skills you have learned in this book. Each new chapter will expand this definition of success until, when you have reached the end of this book, it will include "life, the universe, and everything."

By narrowly restricting your definition of success at this point, you will be able to structure your day for success, rather than for failure. Usually, no matter how well some Deadly Dieters do, they are never satisfied because "it could be better." This thought becomes a vicious cycle that never allows you to enjoy the fruits of your labor. It is important that you immediately get on a new success cycle and off the old failure cycle.

Success Journal

Date	Success

By compiling a list of successes NO MATTER HOW SMALL, you begin to build up a track record that will become useful later on. At some point down the road, when you have a setback, you will have to contend with many negative thoughts. One of them will be, "I have made no progress and am right back where I started." Of course, this will not be true. But when you are having a setback, it is hard to see anything positive. By reading your Success Journal, you will be able to effectively counteract this negative and destructive thinking.

The success table can be used as an example for your Success Journal. This is the most difficult exercise in the book because it is the easiest to forget. You can remember by making several dozen copies of a master and putting them in a cheap three-ring binder. Place this binder on your pillow and its location will remind you to make an entry prior to going to sleep. After writing in your Success Journal, place the binder on your night stand. In the morning, after you make the bed, place the binder back on your pillow.

Skills Checklist

The following skills will need to be practiced on a daily basis. This checklist will be placed at the end of each chapter to help you remember the skills you need to practice.

☐ Identify stress levels

☐ Natural Breathing

☐ Progressive Relaxation (15 muscle groups)

☐ Mental Imagery

☐ Coping with a panic attack

☐ Morning ritual (Take Time To Live)

☐ Evening ritual (Success Journal)

3

Sources of Stress

Great gains are not won except by great risks.
—HERODOTUS, 480 B.C.

You are now ready to begin the prevention method for stress reduction. Stress comes from within your own mind. Worry, negative thinking, cognitive distortions are all reasons for becoming stressed. What I will do for you in this chapter is point out five very significant sources of stress in the life of the Deadly Dieter. There are certainly more mental sources of stress than these five. These, however, tend to be common to most people whose lives are ruled by the Deadly Diet. These five stressors not only make you feel uncomfortable, but can also keep you from beginning to make positive changes in your life.

The first of these mental stressors is an unawareness of personal rights. Many Deadly Dieters are surprised to hear that they have basic rights such as happiness and joy. For instance, when they cause pain to themselves by vigorous exercise, they don't realize that life, for them, can be any better.

2.   Second, many Deadly Dieters tend to relinquish personal responsibility for their actions and their lives in general. The Deadly Dieter usually feels totally responsible for those around her, but feels very little responsibility for herself, often hoping that others will care for her.

3.   A third mental stressor is making decisions based upon unreasonable expectations. Deadly Dieters commonly expect to be perfect; they expect happiness through thinness; and they expect that other people won't like them unless they are not "fat."

The stressful behavior of owning other people's problems is why the Deadly Dieter is seen as such a "nice" person. Getting her needs met is very difficult for the person with a Deadly Diet. Since she has no rights, she spends very little time being "selfish" and considerable time doing for others at her own expense.

4.   Finally, taking risks is very rare for Deadly Dieters. They invariably describe themselves as people who value safety and security. Without a doubt the biggest risk that the person is unwilling to take is that of gaining weight, even if only a few pounds or ounces.

Your task in this chapter will be to identify and understand these mental stressors.

Forgetting Your Rights

The last twenty years have focused attention on individual rights and how important it is to stand up for them. The civil rights movement, the women's rights movement, and the gay rights movement are a few of the resulting cultural upheavals our society has experienced. Our constitution guarantees us certain "inalienable rights," and it is important to accept the fact that all humans do have certain basic human rights—even you!

People with Deadly Diets are generally keenly aware of other people's rights, while tending to ignore their own. I am not sure why this is so, but I suspect that it has to do with a distorted view of "selfishness." You may be very concerned that others do not perceive you as a self-centered and selfish individual. But this concern for others may blind you to some very basic rights of your own.

Ignoring or forgetting your rights can be a strong source of stress. Rights are given to you by birth. Your recognition of a right is called a "need." Expression of this need/right is a "want." When you obtain one of these wants, you behave assertively. But when you do not act according to your wants, or express your needs, or recognize your rights, life can be very stressful. In such a situation, people often breathe improperly, tense their muscles, and allow their minds to race.

When this occurs, you have once again begun the spinning of the Control Cycle. Your distorted thinking regarding your rights leads to stress. You either don't eat or binge to make yourself feel better. Denial of your rights is a sure way to be out of control.

In his marvelous book, *The Art of Selfishness*, David Seabury points out that you cannot solve your personal problems until you accept your own basic rights with energy and conviction. Constructive selfishness does not exclude consideration of others. Rather, it is used to protect and foster your own emotional growth. Once you understand that what is best for you is ultimately best for other people, you can allow yourself the freedom to make constructive choices concerning the quality of your life. Seabury describes a person who has a healthy selfishness: "You allow yourself time to think, to decide, to develop. You seek the larger ends and the broader services, and from a respect for your own nature, you protect yourself against others."

Denial of self has been a philosophy for many groups of people throughout the ages and has often been upheld as a supreme form of goodness. Yet, the martyrdom that generally results from such a view of life is a caricature of healthy selflessness. The morality of self-denial offers only two alternatives: either total self-abnegation or thoughtless greed. But neither of these extremes are necessary or helpful. Seabury pleads for a more moderate alternative: a middle course between "ruthless riot and rigid regulation."

The distinction between destructive selfishness and constructive selfishness is important for you to remember. Constructive selfishness means you take care of yourself *before* taking care of others. Destructive selfishness means taking care of yourself *instead* of taking care of others. Being constructively selfish doesn't mean not caring about others. It is not a matter of whether you help others, but *when you help them.*

Your right to protect and take care of yourself and your right to consider your own needs is absolutely essential to being a healthy functioning human being. You cannot give to others unless you have nurtured and taken care of yourself. It is impossible to draw water from an empty well. A starving person hasn't the strength to feed others. Sacrifice and martyrdom are the bricks that pave the road to psychological malnutrition.

Near the end of his book, Seabury proposes a New Bill of Rights in order to protect a person's selfhood. The following two lists have been adapted from his suggestions and those in *The Relaxation & Stress Reduction Workbook*. Read them over carefully and notice your own reactions to each of the items.

My Rights as a Human Being

1. **I HAVE THE RIGHT** to protect and warm my body.

2. **I HAVE THE RIGHT** to put myself first, sometimes.

3. **I HAVE THE RIGHT** to drink—the quenching of thirst.

4. **I HAVE THE RIGHT** to avoid injury and sickness.

5. **I HAVE THE RIGHT** to make mistakes and be responsible for them.

6. **I HAVE THE RIGHT** to rest and to repair my body.

7. **I HAVE THE RIGHT** to eat according to my constitution.

8. **I HAVE THE RIGHT** to protect my privacy.

9. **I HAVE THE RIGHT** to choose my own marriage partner.

10. **I HAVE THE RIGHT** to love and nurture—to give and to get.

11. **I HAVE THE RIGHT** to joy—to play and refresh my strength.

12. **I HAVE THE RIGHT** to work according to my talents.

13. **I HAVE THE RIGHT** to think and feel according to my convictions.

14. **I HAVE THE RIGHT** to be judged by all I am, and do in a decade rather than by a single action.

15. **I HAVE THE RIGHT** to make my own friends.

16. **I HAVE THE RIGHT** to change my mind or decide on a different course of action.

17. **I HAVE THE RIGHT** to protest unfair treatment or criticism.

18. **I HAVE THE RIGHT** to negotiate for change.

19. **I HAVE THE RIGHT** to ask for help or emotional support.

20. **I HAVE THE RIGHT** to ignore the advice of others.

21. **I HAVE THE RIGHT** to be illogical in making decisions.

22. **I HAVE THE RIGHT** not to have to justify myself to others.

23. **I HAVE THE RIGHT** to choose not to respond to a circumstance.

24. **I HAVE THE RIGHT** not to take responsibility for someone else's problems.

25. **I HAVE THE RIGHT** to be appreciated as a person in my own right, not considered as an appendage or extension of someone else.

26. **I HAVE THE RIGHT** to be acknowledged as a person who contributes to society, no matter how small that contribution might be.

27. **I HAVE THE RIGHT** not to justify my behavior to others.

28. **I HAVE THE RIGHT** to say: "I don't know," "I don't understand," "I don't care," and "No!"

29. **I HAVE THE RIGHT** to waste time.

30. **I HAVE THE RIGHT** to be happy!

[*Adults Only*]

A. **I HAVE THE RIGHT** to freedom—for experimental living.

B. **I HAVE THE RIGHT** to decide my own responsibilities.

C. **I HAVE THE RIGHT** to set my own standards.

D. **I HAVE THE RIGHT** to make and act upon my own decisions.

E. **I HAVE THE RIGHT** to the fulfillments of sex.

F. **I HAVE THE RIGHT** to develop my beliefs of good and bad, right and wrong, free of conventional pressure.

G. **I HAVE THE RIGHT** to a constructive expression of every facet of my personality.

H. **I HAVE THE RIGHT** to refuse coercion as a means of determining my conduct.

I. **I HAVE THE RIGHT** to develop without regard to "rules" so long as society is not injured.

Some of these rights may offend your sensibilities or your value system. For example, if you have been brought up to believe that there is only one way of thinking about the world and that all other ways are bad and wrong, number 13 or letter F may seem morally wrong to you.

But these rights are not meant to contradict your own ethical principles. If you look at them carefully, you may discover that they are even more fundamental than many of your own values. For example, you may have been raised to believe in a Supreme Being as the only explanation for understanding the universe. Underlying that belief is a more basic right: the right to choose to believe in a Supreme Being whether or not other people pressure you to accept or reject this idea.

One of your most basic rights is to care for yourself—even the Bible says you were created in the image of God. If this is part of your belief system, then it is important to realize that one of your most important functions in life is to care for yourself. By acknowledging your own rights, you can begin to consistently engage in self-care activities that tend to nourish you emotionally. The more you can exercise this right, the less time you will spend in doing things that bring about psychological malnutrition.

You must remember that human beings cannot *force* other people to think a certain way. We can influence each other and try to bring people around to our way of thinking, but the ultimate choice to accept or reject something always lies with the individual. Accepting your rights means that *you* make choices. These choices are the expression of your uniqueness as an individual.

Running From Responsibility

Any discussion of individual rights must be followed by the concept of responsibility. Unfortunately, the word "responsibility" has begun to lose its meaning because so many people use it as a way of manipulating others. By insisting that another person be "responsible," we often really mean that we want the person to behave in a way pleasing to ourselves.

Most people understand responsibility as taking the initiative for what needs to be done, following through on a promise, or doing what is the "right" thing. You will notice that all of these definitions focus on behavior. I would like to expand this a bit and include the consequence of behavior as well in the definition of "responsibility."

My definition of responsibility is *being willing to accept the consequences of your behavior without blame or excuse.* Although most people pay lip service to this idea in our society, in practice it is not a popular habit. Many people try very hard to separate their behavior from its consequences. As Americans, we believe in rugged individualism and therefore think it is our right to make decisions without taking the consequences into account. In other words, we are willing to accept our behavior, but are not willing to accept its consequences. Everybody wants to drive faster than 55, but nobody wants the ticket. There are two basic reasons for this dilemma: societal models and poor professional advice.

Many of the public individuals who influence our thinking and behavior tend to act as if there is a natural separation between behavior and consequences. For example, even though most politicians are honest and upright, the ones we tend to hear about are those who engage in disreputable behavior. And when was the last time you read or heard of a public official caught with his fingers in the till who admitted full responsibility for his behavior? Other highly visible people such as upper-level executives in corporations or popular entertainers also make the news when engaged in some type of questionable behavior. More often than not, we are fed a litany of excuses and alibis for why the person is not responsible for what happened.

The second major reason that people tend to blame others and excuse their own behavior is because of the bad advice that the professional mental health community has given the public. My profession has tended to hand people excuses on a silver platter—teaching us that it is okay to blame others or dig up alibis for our behavior. Responsibility has been conspicuously absent from the vocabulary of the professional therapist for too many years. It is time now for therapists to accept the fact that people can learn how to be responsible for what they do. And if people choose not to be responsible, then it is society's right to deal with the behavior according to its laws.

My profession has always enjoyed sticking labels on people. We have seemed more secure when we have been able to find the "correct" pigeonhole for our clients. Labels like *schizophrenic, hysteric, neurotic, borderline,* and *anorectic* are just a few of the many categories we have at our disposal. The problem is that labels can have a powerful negative influence on the people unfortunate enough to receive them. First of all, they catch the therapist up in a vicious cycle of explaining nothing at all about the particular problem. "Why doesn't that person eat?" "Because she has anorexia." "How do you know she has anorexia?" "Because she doesn't eat." Labels also have a negative influence in the community. Whether you are labelled as "thin" or "anorectic" will determine how people will react to you. Finally, labels are wonderful excuses. Years ago, when I worked in a private mental hospital, one of the residents escaped from the grounds and took his clothes off in the middle of a busy street. He then sat down and stopped traffic. When he was brought back inside, I overheard a staff member ask him why he had behaved so. His answer: "Because I'm a paranoid schizophrenic."

Another "psychological" excuse is frequently used with small children. If a parent who has a problem with a small child takes that child to a pediatrician, the parent may be told not to worry because the child is "just going through a stage and will soon outgrow it." I have even heard children tell adults to leave them alone because the child was just going through a stage. The surprising thing is that this tends to work—the adult backs off. In fact, it has worked so well with kids that adults are just now beginning to recognize stages of growth during adulthood. Books have been written describing these stages, and adults have transformed what is now called the "mid-life crisis" into an excuse of their own. This means that at some time in his or her thirties or forties a person can act totally irresponsible while telling those around him that it is "just a stage." "Not to worry, I'll be back to normal in a couple of years."

Describing these concepts as excuses does not imply that we are dealing with false or mythical ideas. There certainly are such things as mental disorders and stages of growth. However, being responsible means that you don't use these abstract concepts to excuse your particular behavior, or to place the blame for what you do on something or someone else.

The Great Expectations

What is an expectation? Very simply, it is something that will probably happen. The opposite of an expectation is a wish—something that will probably not happen. An expectation is a mirror of reality; a wish is a mirror of fantasy. Neither of these is better or worse than the other. As mature human beings, we all need to have a firm grip on reality while simultaneously enjoying the freedom of an active fantasy life.

Many Deadly Dieters attempt to convert their wishes into expectations. Have you ever wished for something so hard that, even though it had little chance of happening, you were disappointed when it didn't? When you treat wishes as expectations, you harbor what is known as "unrealistic expectations."

Wishes and unrealistic expectations are the same thing—fantasy events. Realistic expectations are their opposite. Unrealistic expectations tend to be wishes pushed to the extreme. Many dieters would be happy to have an acceptable figure; the Deadly Dieter will not be happy until she has the perfect figure. The Deadly Dieter's wishes are similar to those of other people, except that the Deadly Dieter's wishes have become converted into expectations.

Not only does the Deadly Dieter confuse reality and add stress to her life by trying to transform wishes into expectations, but she is also influenced by the Great American Getting Game. If the American mentality could be summed up in one word, it would be the word "get." If a person can't get success, popularity, sex appeal, an ideal figure, endless peace, a suburban house, or a perfect mate, then something is terribly wrong.

We often feel we must frantically get something extreme in order to feel peace and happiness. It is that very attitude—one of *tremendous* expectations of ourselves and of an unreal world—that makes us miserable, ill, and fearful. We have put our sights on an unreachable goal. This particular American myth is a deathtrap, and its overblown expectations are nothing more than poison in disguise. The key is to put up a permanent barrier between your wishes and your expectations. Although there is nothing wrong with wishing for something you can't have, it is essential to recognize that the wish is just fantasy and nothing more. When you can correctly identify your desires as either unrealistic wishes or realistic expectations, you will begin to reduce the pain and frustration in your life.

"If only I could get, get, get." Endless disappointment and perceptions of deprivation and pain are the price you pay if you want to participate in the getting game.

And so many of your expectations get piled right back on top of you! You think you should please and perform for others in order to feel good about yourself. You think you should act a certain way around people you know. You think you should be more attractive and tip the scales at the perfect weight. Or you think you should never say anything that would hurt someone's feelings. And the faintest sign of someone else's disapproval comes as a mortal blow.

To let go of unrealistic expectations is to live in the instant. It means dumping your old value system, releasing your fearful hold on the past and future, and living for the moment—a moment in which the past cannot touch you and the future is but a dream and need not be feared.

Robert had been one of the few male clients on the Deadly Diet to come to the clinic. His bulimia had lasted for six years when he finally decided to call it quits. He discovered that he had paid a severe price for trying to pursue the American dream: a severe case of fear and depression. For years, his life was ruled by a series of dictatorial "if onlys": "If only I had that perfect girlfriend that would make me feel good. If only I was athletic and more popular. If only I could get that special something—whatever it is—that would make me happy like everybody else, then life would be grand, and I would be happy all the time." Extreme? Of course. But Robert believed every word of it.

He always believed that if he wasn't loved, popular, or held in perfect admiration by the world, then life was a big zero. His expectations were incredibly high and unobtainable. But during his moments of discomfort and bouts of depression, his unrealistic expectations all seemed perfectly reasonable.

Strangely enough, Robert often had more people in his life than some of his buddies did. But many times it still felt like the social life he had just wasn't enough. He began to feel the urge of needing a bigger "love fix," more approval, more love, more peace, more, more, more of everything. Unfortunately, the more he sought, the less he got.

Eventually he realized how stressful these unrealistic expectations and wishes were on his life. After several months in therapy, Robert learned how to identify and challenge these mental stressors. Even in the depths, Robert began to find the mental strength to challenge his craziness. He began to notice that some of his happiest friends weren't popular or loved constantly. Many of them lived alone with a social calendar one-tenth of his. And yet they seemed so content. Robert began to think that their contentment might have come about because they knew the difference between healthy, natural, realistic desires and tyrannical, deadly, sky-high expectations.

Robert began to back off, and things began to flow naturally. Love and peace came unannounced and on their own, without his begging and pleading. They were merely by-products of letting go. He didn't have to strive, obtain, or work at anything. It was all just a matter of setting his sights on the moment.

Once he was able to release such enormous stresses from his life, Robert found that the urge to binge was beginning to decrease. He was also able to learn even more skills for dealing with his binge behavior and his emotional depressions.

You are probably saying, "It just sounds too easy," or "I can't think like that." But it is easy—and yet so very hard for you if you have been programmed to get, get, get, and despair over why you haven't gotten that magic, unobtainable stuff. In Robert's case, that stuff was love, peace, and popularity. Little by little, he began to let go of those deadly expectations. Now, during times when he actively works at doing this—by letting go of the fear of missing out—he suddenly feels content and peaceful, regardless of who he is with, where he is at, or what he is doing.

One of the ways that you can tell whether or not you are dealing with unrealistic expectations is how often you play the "if onlys." An "if only" always uses the formula "If only A, then B." Here are a few "if onlys" that might ring a bell for you.

- If only I was that perfect weight—then things would be marvelous.

- If only I could just find love—a mate, sex, intimacy, closer friendships—then I would be happy and feel so good all of the time.

- If only I could be more successful—a better student, more money, a better career, more things, a better house, travel—then life would be so fulfilling.

- If only I could get to that stage of life where I could just cruise—then I'd have it made.

Exercise

To help you reduce stress in your own life, you might want to find out how strongly you play the Getting Game. Using the "If only . . . then . . ." formula, try to find out how you convert your wishes into unrealistic expectations.

1. If only _____

   then _____

2. If only _____

   then _____

3. If only _____

   then _____

Taking on Monkeys

Even though we all have problems, Deadly Dieters tend to act as if they owned all of the problems belonging to those around them. If someone is feeling sad, the Deadly Dieter will immediately take it upon herself to make that person feel better. Of course, by taking on everyone else's problem, it is then easier to deny or conveniently forget the problem of the Deadly Diet. Helping others is a means for not dealing with one's own problems.

In our society, people are often raised to believe that they aren't supposed to put themselves before others. Women, especially, have been taught that they must take care of others first. If there happen to be any crumbs left over on the table after the banquet, then they might be allowed to have something for themselves. Taking on the problems of others can be a very stressful activity. Not only do you have your own life to contend with, you also have the lives of others. You end up with no time left over to deal with your own problems and needs.

Problems are universal—everyone has them. In 1974, an article in the *Harvard Business Review* suggested that since problems can have a way of tenaciously clinging to us, regardless of how we try to shake them loose, we might as well think of them as the monkeys they resemble. All of us respond to these "monkeys" in different ways.

Maybe you have found that you are so softhearted that you hate to see these monkeys mistreated, starved, or even left alone. Although monkeys are generally uncomfortable and annoying, maybe you at least feel a familiarity toward them that offers your life a certain amount of predictability.

Or maybe you have learned to be a monkey martyr and spend much of your life collecting extra monkeys from other people. Some Deadly Dieters have become so adept at collecting monkeys that they run full-time monkey farms. Unfortunately, when you play the role of a monkey farmer, you usually end up feeling worse and worse with each monkey added to your collection.

Let me give you a good example of a monkey common among Deadly Dieters. In a situation, you find yourself not doing or saying something because doing so might "hurt someone's feelings." The person with the potentially hurt feelings has a monkey that you readily accept. It is imperative that you begin to distinguish between your behavior and other people's feelings. You are *not* responsible for other people's feelings. You *are* responsible for your behavior, thoughts, and feelings. This means that everyone else is also responsible for his or her own behavior, thoughts, and feelings.

If you look closely, you will observe that in many groups, such as families, there are so many monkeys running around loose that it is sometimes difficult to find the owner of these strays. As a collector, rather than finding the owner and firmly giving the monkey back to its proper care-taker, you just pick it up and carry it around until either you or the monkey dies.

Believe it or not, some people even get anxious when they have no monkeys and others do. These people always walk around bent at the waist waiting for somebody's monkey to jump on their back so that they, too, can have a monkey just like everybody else.

If you are tired of having too many monkeys on your back, you need to discover more clearly which monkeys do not belong to you and who tends to give them away to you. The following exercise will help you learn more about this skill of *problem ownership*.

Exercise

For one week keep a daily log of all your significant interactions with other people. Be ready to answer the following questions about each interaction.

1. Did the person directly ask me to do something?

2. Did the person infer that I should or should not have done something?

3. Did I assume that something had been or was being asked or requested of me?

4. Did I meet his or her expectations? How did that make me feel?

5. Did I disappoint that other person?

6. How did that make me feel?

7. Whose problem was it? The other person's or mine?

Living Safely

The Deadly Diet is one of the world's greatest cocoons. It is safe and familiar and totally inaccessible to outsiders. The longer you have been on the Deadly Diet, the more difficult it can be for you to leave its security. From inside, it seems like the biggest risk you can take is to give up the Deadly Diet. Yet avoiding this risk is the most fearful thing you can think of doing.

Almost every Deadly Dieter I have ever known has at some point admitted tremendous fear of the Great Abyss—and overcoming it is often the first great step for many Deadly Dieters. When you begin to contemplate a life without the Deadly Diet, you begin to believe that you will be falling into a great unknown abyss, a vast chasm which is terrifying and dangerous. The Deadly Diet has been like all things you are familiar with—safe, comfortable, predictable, and secure. How can you be sure that your new life will have any of these qualities? You believe that to give up the Deadly Diet is to die an emotional death, to make yourself vulnerable to something larger than yourself. On top of this is the fear that once you have made a commitment to recover, the decision is irreversible. You may be telling yourself, "What if I make a mistake and there really is nothing better than the Deadly Diet?"

Since these concerns halt you cold in your tracks, let's take some time to see the truth of the matter. The truth is that there is no abyss, no void for you to fall into. The void is a black curtain constructed by your fears. And when the curtain is parted, you will enter into a new and beautiful life. When you dare to penetrate the blackness ahead of you, you will be parting the curtain and will see green grass and blue sky. You have believed that life is death; I want you to know that death (to the Deadly Diet) is life.

Your other fear is that you might be mistaken about the possibility of a better life. Believe me, if you make a mistake, you can always turn back. If you really find that life without the Deadly Diet is not for you, it will be easy to come back to this lifestyle.

What I am asking you to do here is to begin to risk. When you risk you become vulnerable, and that is why many people refuse to take risks. But why do you have to take risks? Why can't you live a nice, safe life without things going wrong? Why do bad things have to happen to you?

Let's face it—things do go wrong in life. Sometimes bad things happen because we humans make mistakes. This makes sense to most of us. But at other times things can go dreadfully wrong quite by accident. Bob Greene, the syndicated columnist, has pointed out that it is these accidental events which don't make sense to us. We have all thought or said that "life is not fair," and this phrase echoes the frustration of having things go wrong in spite of our best efforts. Things that go wrong can be trivial or significant—a torn shoelace or death. Take that darkest extreme: no matter how hard we try, death can strike us for the most improbable reasons. In fact, we don't have to do anything wrong to die; we don't have to be careless or foolish or lacking in judgment. It doesn't even have to be our fault.

All of us living in this nuclear age know deep down how terribly fragile the fabric of society really is. Something can go wrong at every turn; we can do our best to maintain our own sanity, but can do nothing about the sanity of others. We build our lives of faith—faith that others will act properly and that nature will act kindly toward us.

Every time we order a meal in a restaurant, we have faith that someone in the kitchen didn't put something deadly in our food. Every time we drive in our car, we have faith that some other driver has not picked us out to help him end his life in a head-on collision. Every time we sleep in a hotel, we have faith that some madman has not planted a bomb in the next room. Every time we fly in an airplane, we have faith that someone in the same plane is not filled with some twisted idea of revenge or personal gain. The scary possibility always exists that our faith has been misguided and we have made some wrong assumptions about other people. Even if we had guarantees about people, we could still get food poisoning, our car's brakes could go out, the hotel could catch on fire, and the airplane could inexplicably crash. Life is an act of faith.

Since we do live in a world based on probability, it is important to recognize this fact. We cause unnecessary problems for ourselves when we begin to demand guarantees for uncertain parts of our lives. Often Deadly Dieters carve out a portion of their existence and demand certitude. "I am not going to change my eating habits unless I can have a guarantee that I won't gain weight." "I will not tell anybody about my eating problem unless I can be absolutely certain they will not ridicule or make fun of me." Since there are no guarantees, at best only extremely high or low probabilities, this kind of thinking puts you in the twilight zone of life.

You have only two options as a human being living in a world that can be confusing and unpredictable. The first is to look for a safe and secure place in which to hide—and eating disorders are great hiding places. The problem arises when the hiding place forces you into a life of ritualistic inflexibility. The stress that results from this choice can be unbearable.

The only other option is to realistically accept the fact that life is necessarily unpredictable and sometimes unsafe. No amount of wishing or denial will change this. To live is to risk. This does not mean that you need to take unnecessary risks or to jeopardize yourself and others with foolish behavior. It means that reasonable caution can allow you to live a life somewhere between certitude and chaos. This fine edge can only be walked if you understand this fact: THERE IS NO CERTAINTY IN LIFE!

If you cannot accept a world governed by probability, then you can only become trapped by the worries of your mind and begin to anticipate events that may never happen. You can even go further and convince yourself that if these awful events did in fact happen, you would be totally incapacitated to deal with them.

This constant worry about what might happen is essentially useless. No amount of worry has ever prevented a misfortune from happening. What if you were afraid that your spouse would run off with someone else? Would your worrying prevent it from happening? Probably the opposite—the constant tension and worry you bring to the relationship might actually help it fall apart.

If you choose the option of living life safely within a supposedly safe cocoon, then you will never realize the joy of going into the sunshine with your newly acquired wings helping you to soar through the fresh air of freedom.

By choosing the second option and recognizing the world of probability, you can learn to live in the present with all its joys and sorrows, hurts and happiness. You can avoid the mind trap of worrying about the future and feeling the misery of always wondering when the impending disaster will hit. The second option puts you back in the mainstream of life and allows you to live it to its fullest.

Faith can certainly be reasonable, but never certain. And because there is no certitude, you can experience the joy of anticipation, the excitement of change, and the wonder of growth.

Exercise

Since there is an element of risk in every human action, including inaction, the question is not whether we should take risks, but which of those risks we choose to take. And this requires a skilled ability to assess the degree of risk in any given activity. To check your ability to accurately assess different risks, study the list of sixteen activities below. Which, in your opinion, are the safer activities, and which are the more dangerous? Assign a value of 1 to the safest activity and a value of 16 to the most dangerous one.

_____ Smoking 1.4 cigarettes
_____ Living two months with a cigarette smoker
_____ Drinking one-half liter of wine
_____ Working one hour in a coal mine
_____ Living two days in Boston
_____ Drinking Miami's water for one year
_____ Living two months in Denver
_____ Traveling six minutes by canoe
_____ Traveling 10 miles by bicycle
_____ Traveling 150 miles by car
_____ Traveling 1,000 miles by jet
_____ Having a chest X-ray
_____ Living next to a nuclear power plant for five years
_____ Eating forty tablespoons of peanut butter
_____ Drinking thirty 12-ounce cans of diet soda
_____ Eating 100 charcoal-broiled steaks

_____ **TOTAL**

As you may have guessed by now, all of the risks on the list, according to physicist Richard Wilson, are equal (Wilson 1979). The risk of getting cancer and heart disease from smoking 1.4 cigarettes is equal to the risk of experiencing a fatal accident during a 10-mile bicycle ride, which is equal to the risk of contracting liver cancer from the aflatoxin B contained in 40 tablespoons of peanut butter. On a statistical basis, each of the sixteen activities on the list will shorten your life by 15 minutes.

Homework

1. Reread the section entitled "Forgetting Your Rights" and answer the following questions:
   a. Which rights do you especially like?
   b. Which were you unaware of?
   c. Which are you aware of but do not exercise?
   d. Which do you think you don't have?

Think about your answers to these questions and other issues related to your rights for an entire day. When you have done this, write down at the end of the day what you have learned about your rights. Try to make your essay at least a page long; longer if you like. When you have completed this assignment, continue on to assignment 2.

2. Reread the section entitled "Running From Responsibility." Answer the following questions:
   a. Are you aware of the consequences to your eating behaviors?
   b. Whom do you tend to blame for what happens to you?
   c. What kind of excuses do you use to justify your behavior?
   d. Are you willing to become more responsible for the consequences of your actions by dropping excuses and blaming?

As with the first assignment, think for an entire day about how you accept responsibility. Let these four questions simmer on the back burner of your mind. At the end of the day, write another essay. The purpose of these essays is to force you to put your thoughts on paper. The transition from mind thoughts to words on paper can be difficult, but it can also be rewarding as you learn new things about yourself. Continue to assignment 3 when finished.

3. Reread the section entitled "The Great Expectations" and answer the following questions:
   a. What are some of your unrealistic expectations?
   b. Which of your wishes tend to turn into expectations?
   c. Which areas of your life are easier for you to be realistic about?
   d. Which of your unrealistic expectations do you want to change?

Again, think about your answers to these questions for about a day. Write down your thoughts about unrealistic expectations. When this assignment is complete, go to assignment 4.

4. Reread the section entitled "Taking on Monkeys." Answer the following questions:
   a. Who tends to want to give you monkeys to care for?
   b. Which type of monkeys do you find hard to resist?
   c. How often do you put others' needs ahead of your own?
   d. What are you planning to do with the monkeys you've been collecting?

Write your thoughts out as you have done for the previous questions.

5. Reread the section entitled "Living Safely" and answer the following questions:
   a. What guarantees do you insist upon?
      Which risks are you unwilling to take in your life?
   b. What does this unwillingness do to your life?
   c. What would happen to you—really!—if you were to take some of these risks?
   d. Which "myths of certitude" are you going to let go of?

Complete the final essay.

6. Now that you have carefully thought about these five universal stressors, it is important that you discover what you have learned from doing all this work. Your next assignment in this chapter will be to read through each essay you have written and write a summary paragraph for each one which answers the following question: "What have I learned about myself from this essay?" When finished, go to assignment 7.

7. We have found, in our work with Deadly Dieters, that unstructured time can cause all sorts of problems. Most of our clients tell us that their eating is worse in the evenings and on weekends. As long as they are busy things work out pretty good. If someone imposes structure on them—whether from work or school—they can often deal with their Deadly Diet more sensibly. Bingers especially find that they are okay as long as they are involved in school, work, personal activities, or appointments. When a block of free time occurs, they tend to gravitate toward the kitchen.

   Learning to structure your day is an extremely important skill for you to learn. Deadly Dieters find it very difficult to accurately budget their time. They find themselves driven to keep busy, either because they feel a sense of duty to be productive or because being busy keeps them from having to deal with the problem. Living one day at a time is one of the major factors in your overcoming the Deadly Diet.

   To help you accomplish this goal, I want you to keep a daily schedule of what you need to do for the day. This is to be done each night before going to bed. Your evening ritual will now include both the completion of your Success Journal and the planning of your daily schedule. It is important to remember that this planning only be done twenty-four hours in advance—one day at a time.

In planning for your daily activities, you need to include several events every day: (1) activities outside your home, (2) anything in your home, (3) homework assignments from this book, and (4) fun. That's right—fun! Deadly Dieters often forget how to enjoy themselves. Since having fun often makes you feel guilty, you can avoid feeling guilty by not having fun. You must plan something fun for yourself every day. Fun means something totally decadent, without any social redeeming value whatsoever. If this means watching a bird out your window, reading a trashy novel, taking a bubble bath, going for a walk, or watching the soaps, so be it. You may include other people in your fun time if you so desire. But remember that it is your fun time—they are merely tagging along for the ride.

As you plan your Daily Schedule, you will learn how to estimate time requirements and become more realistic as to how much you can expect of yourself in a typical day. Consequently, your first week or so may be quite ragged as you learn to work out the bugs in your daily planning.

Finally, you will want to follow the four guidelines below for daily schedule planning. Many people make their planning more difficult by violating these four rules. In order to make your daily schedule work, you need to make your daily goals:

a. *Positive.* Too often people set negative goals. "Today I will not binge." Each of your daily goals needs to be stated in positive terms.

b. *Specific.* Many goals are too vague in nature such as "Today I will try harder." The more specific the goals, the easier it will be to reach them.

c. *Measurable.* Goals are more easily reachable when they use time and space limitations. How long will you do it? Where will you do it?

d. *Reasonable.* People with eating disorders tend to set highly unrealistic goals for themselves. This, of course, sets up a negative failure cycle. By setting reasonable daily goals, you change that cycle to a positive success-oriented cycle.

Once you have structured your time for the following day, there are two rules you must follow. (1) You must do whatever is on the daily schedule. (2) If you don't want to, then change it. These two rules may sound contradictory, but they really are not. The important point is that you learn to control time. Since you want to have structure but also need to be flexible, both of these rules work to complement each other. If something comes up that is not on your daily schedule, then erase it, put in the new activity, and follow through.

Using a daily schedule has two parts: writing it down and doing it. The first is the most important of the two. If you are having trouble at first following the schedule, don't worry. Just keep making it each evening. If your goal is to follow the schedule perfectly, then you will only do this assignment for a day or two before giving up because you couldn't do it perfectly. However, if your goal is merely to fill out the schedule, then you will continue the assignment whether or not you have been able to follow the schedule. It is more important for you now to complete the schedule rather than follow it. The second part will come later.

8. You can now begin to speed up your muscle relaxation by working on only seven muscles instead of the fifteen you have been using. This shortened progressive relaxation should only take about ten minutes. The following dialogue may be taped and played the first time you use this shortened method.

Shortened Relaxation

Begin by concentrating all of your attention on your RIGHT HAND and ARM. Hold your right arm straight out in front of you, with your elbow bent just slightly, and make a fist. Try to tense not only the muscles of your hand and lower arm, but also the bicep at the same time. Hold the tension. . . . Now relax your arm and let it gently fall to the side. Feel the relaxation take over your entire right arm. Already your breathing has begun to slow down and you are beginning to feel relaxed and calm.

Keeping your right arm completely relaxed, let's do the same thing with your LEFT HAND and ARM. Tense it tightly so that you feel those tense muscles from your shoulder all the way down to your fingers. . . . Relax those muscles and let your left arm and hand become perfectly limp and relaxed. Notice how both of your arms are now completely relaxed. . . . You are able to notice the relaxation begin to come over your entire body. . . . Your breathing has slowed way down. . . . You are feeling calm and peaceful.

The next muscle group will consist of the many small muscles in your FACE and SCALP. You are going to do several different things all at the same time. First, wrinkle up your forehead so the top of your head is all tight and wrinkly. Next, squint your eyes. Now, wrinkle up your nose, bite down, and finally pull the corners of your mouth back. Feel this tension throughout your entire face and scalp. . . . Now, relax and feel that wonderful relaxation flowing throughout your entire face and scalp. . . . Feel all the tension draining away as the muscles in your face become loose and relaxed. . . . Feel the skin becoming smooth and soft.

Next, bend your head forward and pull your chin downward toward your chest without actually touching your chest. In other words, I want you to counterpose the muscles in the front part of the NECK against those in the back of your neck. You will feel just a little bit of shaking or trembling in these muscles as you tense them. Study that tension. . . . Okay, relax your neck and throat and put your head back in a comfortable position. . . . Enjoy the peaceful relaxation you now feel throughout your throat, neck, face, and scalp.

Next, I want you to concentrate on the large muscles in your UPPER TORSO—the muscles in your shoulders, back, chest, and stomach. Again, you will do several different things at the same time. First, take a really deep breath and hold it. While doing this, pull your shoulder blades back and together. Now make your stomach as hard as you can. Try to feel that tension in every muscle. . . . Relax everything and completely let go of all the tension in your upper body. . . . Experience the utter calm and peacefulness of relaxation from your stomach to the top of your head.

Next, focus your attention on your RIGHT THIGH, CALF, and FOOT. Lift your right leg up, straighten out your knee, and pull your toes up toward your face. Experience the tension in your entire leg. . . . Let go and completely relax your leg and foot. . . . Notice how pleasant you now feel all over.

Finally, do the same thing with your LEFT LEG, creating as much tension as you can from your toes to your hip. Make your entire leg and foot tense, hard, and tight. . . . Now, relax and feel the warm glow of relaxation starting at the top of your head and spreading gently through your body down to the tips of your toes.

9. To make your mind-calming imagery even more realistic, you can make full use of your five senses during the scene. Try to actually see things in your imagination, hear things, see, taste, and touch a variety of experiences in your world. The following scene—adapted from the book, *Hypnosis and Behavior Modification: Imagery Conditioning*, by Kroger and Fezler—is a good example of the kind of scene you can develop for your own use. You can use this scene with your new seven-step muscle relaxation procedure.

Imagery Scene

I am walking along the beach; it is mid-July. It is very, very warm. It is 5:00 in the afternoon. The sun has not yet begun to set, but it is getting low on the horizon. The sun is a golden blazing yellow, the sky a brilliant blue, the sand a dazzling, glistening white in the sunlight. I can feel the cold, wet, firm, hard-packed sand beneath my feet As I deeply inhale, I can smell the salt in the air. There is a residue of salt deposited on my lips from the ocean spray. I can taste it if I lick my lips. I can hear the beating of the waves. The rhythmic lapping to and fro of the water against the shore. Now I can hear the far-off cry of a distant gull as I continue to walk.

Suddenly I come to a sand dune, a mound of pure white sand. Covering the mound are bright yellow buttercups, deep pink moss roses. I sit down on its crest and look out to sea. The sea is like a mirror of silver reflecting the sun's rays, a mass of pure white light, and I am gazing intently into this light. As I continue to stare into the sun's reflection off the water, I begin to see flecks of violet, darting spots of purple intermingling with the silver. Everywhere there is silver and violet. There is a violet line along the horizon; a violet halo around the flowers.

Now the sun is beginning to set. With each movement, with each motion of the sun into the sea, I become deeper and deeper relaxed. The sky is turning crimson, scarlet, pink, amber, gold, and finally orange as the sun sets.

I am now engulfed in a deep purple twilight, a velvety blue haze. I look up to the night sky. It is a brilliant starry night. I am vaguely aware of the beating of the waves, the smell and taste of the salt, the sea, the sky. And I feel myself carried upward and outward into space, one with the universe.

Skills Checklist

☐ Forgetting your rights: exercise and essay

☐ Running from responsibility: essay

☐ The great expectations: exercise and essay

☐ Taking on monkeys: exercise and essay

☐ Living safe: exercise and essay

☐ Five summary paragraphs

☐ Daily schedule

☐ Shortened relaxation

☐ Continue Natural Breathing as needed

☐ Mental imagery (use more sensory detail)

☐ Morning rituals (add "My Rights as a Human Being")

☐ Evening rituals (add the daily schedule)

4

Voice Training

Nothing in the affairs of men is worth worrying about.
—PLATO, c. 375 B.C.

People with eating disorders tend to be chronic worriers. Being a good worrier is something you must practice and develop, because it is an acquired skill—you are not born with it. You probably began worrying at an early age by imitating another worrier. Practice was often tacitly encouraged, until today you have become a master worrier who reflexively starts catastrophizing with the first awareness of danger.

Below are some typical statements that worriers tend to use. Check off those that sound like you.

☐ I can't stand this any longer.

☐ These feelings are dangerous and could hurt me.

☐ I am a bad person because I did that.

☐ I shouldn't have done that (*or* I should do this).

☐ That person is terrible because he did that to me.

☐ If that should happen to me, it would be a tragedy.

☐ Whenever I enter a crowded room people always look at me.

☐ If only things were different, I could be happy.

☐ Why can't I make myself change?

☐ Everybody can do things better than I can.

Worry saps your energy, stresses your body, forces you to live with destructive emotions, and makes you an unhappy person. As Charles Mayo once said, "Worry afflicts the circulation, the heart, the glands, the whole nervous system." There is a direct relationship between how much you worry and how unhappy you are.

It is not necessary to worry. You only do it out of habit because you learned it long ago. Worriers often justify this habit by saying that not to worry is to show a lack of concern. They also appear puzzled when questioned about the significance of worry. "After all, if I didn't worry about things, I couldn't solve or avoid problems."

But there are major differences between worry and *concern*. Both are thinking events, but while worry focuses on the problem (its danger, its painful effects), concern focuses on solutions and strategies to avoid or solve the problem. Worry also tends to attach itself to problems that are beyond the worrier's control, while concern implies a realistic assessment of what can be done and how to do it. As a result, worry tends to drag on without solution until exhaustion or distraction. Concern continues only as long as a solution seems possible.

The key here is to remember that in any given situation we may or may not be able to do anything about it. Sometimes we *are* powerless and unable to make changes. At other times we may feel weak, but are really able to make changes in a difficult situation. In either case, we can lapse into worry by either spending mental energy on situations that *cannot* be changed or by failing to consider the choices we do have in a situation that *can* be changed.

You can stop being a helpless victim of the worry habit. The three steps to conquering worry are (1) awareness, (2) learning, and (3) practice. When you are aware of your own power, you can begin to see how destructive and nonproductive worry actually is. Once you are aware of your power, you can then use the skills in this chapter and succeeding ones to begin the process of controlling your worry. It will then be necessary for you to spend considerable time practicing your new skills in a variety of settings. Practice makes perfect.

Worry does not just happen to you, nor is it an independent force that can control you against your will. YOU must *decide* to worry. Worry cannot be present unless you decide to let it happen. All worriers give away their power to be in charge of their lives. Now is the time to recapture that power.

This power is the power to make choices. You make hundreds of choices every day—some are good choices, some not so good. You choose what to wear, what to eat, what to do in your free time. All of your waking hours are used to make continual choices. In fact, when you think of all the essential trivial choices that you make every day, you can begin to realize how important choices really are. Getting dressed is a fairly insignificant choice. How do you pick out the clothes you are going to wear? Which piece of clothing do you put on first? Which clothes go with which other clothes? Which are appropriate for the temperature? Which will make you comfortable? Which will make you look good?

The availability of choice is like electricity. It is always there, but you can only use it if you choose to turn on the switch. Unless you decide to actually plug into electricity's power, it does you no good, no matter how much of it is there. Worriers selectively turn on the power switch, but usually not often enough. It is important to identify the many different ways you hesitate to use your built-in power source.

When you have become aware of the self-defeating ways that hold you back from using your own built-in power, you can begin to learn how to reprogram yourself for success. You can learn how to be responsible for yourself and to eliminate worry from your life.

Changing Your Thoughts

Your only defense against debilitating emotions is to remember and act on the following principle: YOUR EMOTIONS ARE CAUSED BY YOUR THOUGHTS. Destructive emotions such as depression and guilt are caused and maintained by destructive thoughts (worry) that you are generally not even aware of. Yet, these "automatic thoughts" exert a powerful influence over the emotions you have. Unfortunately, uncovering these destructive thoughts can lead to two major problems.

The first problem occurs when you really begin hearing all of the destructive thinking inside your head. To move from a diffuse awareness of "worrying about things" to a minute awareness of *everything* you worry about can be overwhelming. And as you begin to realize how painful that internal struggle is, you also become aware of a "something" that holds you back from changing your behavior. Many people on the Deadly Diet report that when they try to make positive changes in their life, it feels as if something is stopping them. They also report feeling compelled to do things they would rather not do. For example, one of the little-known facts about people with bulimia is the high incidence of shoplifting, even among those with plenty of money.

One of the most common experiences of Deadly Dieters is the feeling that there is a struggle going on inside between the "good and the bad." You probably view your own internal struggle with equally serious concern. You may even secretly wonder if this conflict is a sign that you are "going crazy." And many therapists would actually treat you as if something was drastically out of kilter if you were to explain the inner dialogue you experience so intensely.

People with feelings like these don't really like to spend a lot of time and effort probing their negative thoughts. Better not to think of them at all. And your intuitions are correct at this point: if you were to suddenly become aware of all your negative, destructive thoughts, you would feel like you had been hit with a tidal wave. Battered by this flood of destructive thoughts, you end up feeling even more overwhelmed, more out of control than before. And maybe even feeling guilty for the damage you're doing to yourself.

Problem number two occurs once you become aware of these destructive thoughts and decide to get rid of them. You find yourself right smack in the middle of a mental riddle: If these destructive thoughts are cluttering up your mind, then how do you use a mind full of destructive thoughts to change your destructive thinking? How do you use a mind stubbornly committed to resisting change to change itself?

To resolve these two problems, I want to teach you a trick. It is a very, very powerful trick, and one that you will be able to use to totally change your thinking.

Begin by imagining that your mind is like a room. As you look through a window into this room, you notice that it is very dingy and dark. It's cluttered and dirty. It's completely uninhabitable. All the dirtiness, all the garbage in this room represents your negative, destructive thinking—your worrying.

Now imagine that this room is all cleaned up. You have cleaned, dusted, swept, and painted, and you have opened the windows to let the sun shine in. And now you see that this mind-room is beautiful, sparkling, bright, and clean—except for a ten-foot pile of garbage right in the middle of the room. You have swept all of the destructive and negative garbage into one pile.

Now imagine a hand reaching inside your room and lifting out the pile of garbage, every last scrap of it, and putting it outside, about a foot or two away. From now on, all of your destructive thinking, all of your worrying, all of your negative thoughts are no longer inside of your head, but rather outside of you—though still very close by. We call the owner of this pile of garbage "the Voice."

The reason we have named it the Voice is very simple. If you've ever been keenly aware of your thinking on a really bad day, you probably had the sensation that there was a voice inside your head talking to you. Although traditional mental health has had a difficult time dealing with this Voice (which, by the way, everybody has), almost everyone recognizes its existence. Most people are also afraid to acknowledge it.

At this point, let us define the Voice. As we said, the Voice is an illusion, it's a trick, it's a pretend game. And yet, it's an illusion that can be quite useful in helping you to make significant changes in your life. The Voice is *the accumulation of all the negative, destructive, worrisome thinking that you've ever been exposed to in your entire life.*

In his book, *The Inner Enemy*, George Bach says that "we must learn to monitor our inner dialogue so that we may see exactly who is talking in there." He then suggests assigning each individual voice a name and enumerating its traits. Our approach is slightly different in that instead of identifying the multiple voices you have, you listen to the Voice that says many things. But Bach's suggestion that we must listen to our internal dialogue is very important. You must be able to identify your enemy before you can fight it.

Perhaps you are asking, "What is so useful about imagining that something exists when it really doesn't?" Well, the answer to this question may lie in the high school algebra that you learned. Mathematicians use a concept called "imaginary numbers." If you remember high school math, you will recall that the square root of -1 does not exist. The square root of -1 is represented by a lower case script i, which stands for an imaginary number, the square root of -1. You may be asking, "What good is it to talk about numbers if they don't really exist?" On the face of it, imaginary numbers don't make any sense. Yet beyond elementary algebra, this imaginary number is essential for studying higher mathematics, engineering, and basic science. It is related to many aspects of contemporary mathematics and physics. These areas of human knowledge all demonstrate that using something imaginary can actually have a practical value. That is exactly what we are doing with the Voice. The Voice does not "really" exist, but the definition that we have given it can make it an extremely powerful tool.

Pretending that the Voice is real will also help you avoid the two pitfalls mentioned earlier: feeling guilty for all your negative thoughts and having to use your negative thoughts to change your negative thoughts. Remember that your Voice is an accident, and you have been victimized by it. You never asked for it; you never took a class in worry skills; you would banish it from your life immediately if you could. It is because of this that you are *not* responsible for its presence. You are, however, responsible for getting rid of it. And that is the intent of Voice Training—to show you how to control the Voice in your life.

I have said that everybody has a Voice. Does that mean that people you know who are happy and seem to have their lives put together have a Voice? The answer is yes. We only differ in terms of how often our individual Voice talks to us, what it may say to us, or how intense it is. Your Voice just happens to be more intense and to speak more frequently than the voices of others. And when people's emotions are running away from them, overwhelming them, or causing pain in their lives, the reason is always because of the actions of their Voice.

You must also realize that you only have *one* Voice—there is not a "good voice" and a "bad voice," with the winner getting to control your life. You *are* the "good" Voice. You represent all those things in your life that are strong, positive, and growth-producing. And it is you who will ultimately defeat the Voice's control of your life.

Even though we know the Voice is fictional, we are going to pretend that it is real. We are going to flesh it out and give it a personality, to talk about its "motives" and "intentions." We will deal with the Voice as if it were a real entity living very close to you at all times. Some people even go so far as to give their voice a name. Some choose to call it Darth Vadar or give it the name of an old boyfriend, girlfriend, or a parent.

As we continue, you will see how useful it is to pretend that the Voice is a real thing. But you must always remember that the Voice is imaginary and that you are real.

Voice training has five phases: (1) Voice Awareness, (2) Voice Analysis, (3) Voice Fighting, (4) Voice Substitution, and (5) Voice Provocation. Each of these phases can best be understood by using an analogy of a garden.

If you were to come back from a long vacation and find your garden dying, the first thing you would need to do would be to become aware of what was causing the destruction of your garden. If it was being destroyed by weeds and you weren't aware of their existence, your garden would continue to die. Even though you knew that your plants were dying, you would have no way of solving the problem. As trivial as it sounds, it would be very important for you to understand the relationship between the weeds and the dying plants. Likewise, you need to be aware of the presence of the Voice in your life. Without Voice Awareness, you will be unable to come up with any practical solutions to your Deadly Diet.

Once you have realized that foreign elements are destroying your garden, you need to carefully analyze each one of them. Each weed will affect your garden differently, just as each Voice message will affect your life. The good gardener will want to classify each weed in order to find the weaknesses in each one. You need Voice Analysis to analyze your Voice's messages and to find the flaws and weaknesses in each one of them.

Once you are aware of the existence of weeds and understand the difference between a weed and a plant, you can begin pulling the weeds up. You can begin taking them out of your garden and stopping the negative effect they have on your plants. Voice Fighting teaches you how to fight back against the Voice. The Voice Fighting procedures you will be learning are quite complex and detailed, but also very powerful and very effective. If you use them consistently, you will find that in a matter of days or weeks significant and profound changes will begin to occur in your life.

Just clearing your garden of weeds will not make the plants in it any healthier. You will still have a garden filled with wilted plants. Your next job is to nurture the plants with water, fertilizer, and plenty of sun. The same holds true for yourself. Voice Substitution teaches you how to nurture yourself: how to encourage the growth of the real you, to become more self-confident, to raise your self-esteem, and to love yourself more.

Some of the techniques you will be using are similar to those often called "the power of positive thinking." Although we owe a lot to the people who have written on this subject, the power of positive thinking by itself is not a very effective technique for people on the Deadly Diet. People who have a severe eating disorder do not do well by just saying positive things to themselves. If you're going to put freshly cut wood into your wood box, it is impossible to do so unless you take the old wood out first. Once you've taken the old wood out, the new wood will fit in quite nicely. The same thing goes for destructive thinking. It is almost impossible to put constructive, positive thoughts in your head if your head is filled with an overwhelming number of destructive, negative thoughts.

Voice Fighting and Voice Substitution work together sequentially. Voice Fighting helps you to push the Voice far enough away from your life that you have room for the nurturing thoughts that you want to put back into your mind. But once the Voice begins to recede from your life, you'll find that there is a mental vacuum. Into this vacuum you must put constructive, positive thoughts so that the Voice does not find it easy to sneak back in. As the Voice begins to leave your room, you want to close the doors and fill up the room with positive, growth-producing thoughts.

The final part of Voice Training is the most difficult and the most lengthy. For some people, Voice Provocation lasts for the rest of their life. If you are watering and nurturing your plants, you very quickly discover that the weeds never went away entirely. Somewhere in the soil are tiny seeds which will sprout more weeds as you feed your plants. The weeds are going to come right back. If you are serious about gardening, you will have to go after them vigorously.

In the same way, you will need to go after the Voice vigorously in order to keep it from coming back into your life. You'll never be able to kill off the Voice entirely. You'll never be able to get rid of it totally. The reason for this is something called human nature: we all have a Voice, and we will have it until the day we die. Therefore you need to take the offensive, rather than stay on the defensive, with the Voice. And you can learn to control the Voice in your life. After all, the issue in your garden is not whether weeds exist, but whether or not you can control these weeds and keep them from affecting your plants. The same holds true for the Voice. The issue is not the presence of the Voice, but who controls your life.

Voice Awareness

Voice Awareness is the foundation upon which you will build the rest of your life-changing skills. It is essential because self-awareness is always a critically important step for moving forward with your life. For instance, if you want to change a habit, such as a nervous tic or smoking, the very first step is to become aware of the habit and how often it occurs.

Of course, the Voice wants just the opposite. Its two most effective weapons are *speed* and *secrecy*. If you don't know about the existence of the Voice or if it is too fast for you, then you will continue to be under its destructive domination.

When the Voice is speaking to you, it is very important to recognize that it is actually talking and to hear *all* that it is saying. The Voice has become such a habit and so constant that you only attend to it during times of stress. In addition, its destructive messages generate destructive emotions that tend to commandeer your attention, preventing you from focusing on the mere words of the Voice's message. Listening to the Voice during times of intense destructive emotions is like trying to watch TV when someone is hitting you on the head with a hammer. Learning to attend to the Voice during these critical times of emotion is a very difficult skill. Yet, it is the very thing you must do in order to have enough information to conquer the Voice.

Words are more powerful than most of us realize. They can affect the way we behave without our being aware of it. They can bury themselves deep within our mind and work to strongly influence us in what we do. We can let the words of other people work on us in such a way that we become slaves to what they say. But even worse, we become slaves to the Voice and its use of certain words and phrases. These words and phrases can be so habitual that we don't even know of their existence.

Many people are hypersensitive to things in their environment such as light, heat, noise, and pollen. There are also people who have a hypersensitivity to the Voice. They are unable to ignore the impact of its words and consequently become victims to their reoccurrence. Does this ever happen to you? Do you ever find yourself being triggered off by what the Voice says? When feeling down, do you find yourself hearing certain words which tend to reinforce your feelings of helplessness, guilt, and depression?

Remember that one of the Voice's best weapons is secrecy. Your task in this first phase of Voice Training is to be able to identify *all* of the things the Voice says to you. This is often difficult because the Voice hides behind its cloak of secrecy by getting you to take ownership of its destructive messages. You have probably said such things as, "I really am stupid," or "I shouldn't hurt people," or "I can't control my eating habits." By making you the owner of destructive messages, the Voice traps you and forces you to abdicate your responsibility for personal growth. The first step in exposing the Voice publicly is to watch your pronouns. Instead of using the "I" pronoun, it is better to translate the phrase so as to turn it into a "you" phrase. "You really are stupid," "You shouldn't hurt people," and "You can't control your eating habits."

Once you have become aware of how often these words are used, you can begin the difficult chore of learning how to stop the Voice from using these words in your presence. You can begin to substitute more constructive words into your everyday vocabulary. Some examples of common destructive Voice phrases are those that begin: *you should, you can't, you'll try,* and *you don't know.*

You should. The phrase "you should" reveals a strong outside influence dictating and judging your actions. "Shoulds" and "have to's" lead to enormous guilt. "You really should stop binging" is a phrase that will make you feel guilty if you are not ready to do so. What you are saying when you use this phrase is, "I don't want to binge like this, but something is forcing me." This "something" is the Voice, which is controlling your life. When you allow the Voice to use words such as "should," "ought," "must," and "have to," you are accepting the fact of being coerced to do something or being kept from doing something you would like to do. One alternative is to replace these words with the phrases "want to" or "choose to." It makes a world of difference. Using the right words can relieve you of the tremendous pressure of being forced to act a certain way.

Say this out loud: "I have to change my eating habits" (or whatever phrase you choose). Now say, "I want to change my eating habits." Did you feel different when you said "want to"? If you did, you are beginning to glimpse what your life will be like when you can regularly defeat the Voice and all its distorted messages. You will begin to find that you can actually have more control over your life.

When you *choose* to do something because you truly want to and not because you are being pressured, you will be able to accept your actions without feeling guilt—even when you make mistakes. You will be making decisions from a position of power. This personal power is yours if you choose it, but drawing on it will take much practice.

You can't. The phrase "you can't" expresses helplessness. It suggests that you wish you could take some action, but that something greater than you is again keeping you from doing what you really want to do. Are any of these statements familiar?

- You can't stand gaining weight.
- You can't take criticism from other people.
- You can't help having panic attacks.
- You can't stand feeling discomfort.

Read these four sentences again and substitute the phrase "I will" or "I choose not to." How does that feel? By using these new words you are forcing yourself to accept personal responsibility for your avoidance behavior. The use of the new phrase will not automatically make you stronger and braver, but it will put the burden of responsibility where it belongs—squarely on your shoulders. You will begin to accept the fact that whatever you do, it is the result of personal choice.

Of course, the mere saying of the words "I will" or "I choose" is no magic incantation. These words will not suddenly allow you to accomplish those things you have been unable to do for years. The critical issue in any situation in which you want to do something but find it difficult to do is whether or not you are actively learning the necessary skills to improve your life. It is much better to say, "I won't change my eating habits yet because the anxiety is too great. However, I am currently working to control my anxiety and am getting better at it every day."

You'll try. The best way to keep yourself from commitment is to insist on *trying*. To try is not necessarily to do. "Trying real hard" is like the exercise wheel in the hamster cage: the animal goes round and round, but never gets anywhere. That is what happens when you merely try. You expend energy, but with no clear conception of specific goals. With no clear goals in mind, it is difficult to determine whether you have succeeded or not.

Many Deadly Dieters have had their problems for so long they are convinced they can't do anything about them. Consequently, they are forever resigned to "trying." When you try, you tell the world, "If I succeed, I will be pleasantly surprised, and if I fail, don't be angry. I never said I would do it."

Don't let the Voice convince you that "trying" is good enough. Instead, begin to use probability estimates. For instance, if you are going to attempt some difficult action, rather than say "I'll try," attempt to estimate how likely you are to succeed in this endeavor. Estimate your chance of success between zero and a hundred percent. If the percentage is too low (less than 75 percent chance of success), then you need to lower your goal and increase your probability. Remember that as you lower your goals, your chances for success go up. And success is the key word, not "proving" your worth by attaining some unrealistic goal.

You don't know. This phrase really means "I don't want to know." If you have knowledge, then you are responsible for what happens. In this sense, ignorance is really bliss. However, you are still responsible for your ignorance. But by saying that you don't know how to change or where to get help, you never really have to change and can blame your problems on the whole world. You can continue for years complaining about your misery and your fears. Here are some familiar examples:

- You don't know what came over you.
- You don't know how to stop binging.
- You don't know what to do about your eating problem.

Do you really want to change? Tell yourself, "I want to know" or "I can find out." Knowledge is everywhere and is yours for the taking. Unfortunately, more knowledge places more demands on your life. With knowledge comes maturity and the ability to make choices, and making choices also requires more energy and personal involvement from you

The following is a structured exercise for you to practice taking more responsibility for the words you use and the words the Voice wants you to use. Take your time in completing the statements and then begin noticing their effect in your everyday conversation.

1. Finish this typical Voice message:
   You should
Now rewrite the sentence so that you are in control.
   I choose/do not choose

2. Finish this typical Voice message:
   You can't

Now rewrite the sentence so that you are in control.
   I will/won't

3. Finish this typical Voice message:
   You can try to

Now rewrite the sentence so that you are in control.

   I have a _____ probability of succeeding
   at_____

4. Finish this typical Voice message:
   You don't know how to

Now rewrite the sentence so that you are in control.
   I want to know how to

As you changed these Voice phrases, did you begin to sense more personal power and more control over your life? If you did, then you need to realize that this is just a glimpse of what it will feel like to completely change your thinking on a regular basis. The Voice Fighting skills that you will learn later will allow you to counter *all* of the messages the Voice throws at you.

Listening to the Voice

Hearing the Voice is not always easy, because listening closely to its messages is an unfamiliar routine for you. To help you become aware of the Voice, you need to become familiar with some of the typical messages it uses on a regular basis. Complete the exercise below by putting an "X" beside any message that your Voice has *ever* said to you. In other words, don't ask yourself whether you believe the statement or not or whether you agree with it. Don't even ask yourself whether your Voice uses this statement frequently. Just look at the statement and then decide whether or not your Voice has *ever* said this to you under any circumstances, at any time.

When you finish this exercise, you may feel as though you have started your autobiography. For the average person with an eating disorder, thirty five out of forty checks is not at all uncommon.

Common Voice Messages
(Adapted from McMullin, Talk Sense to Yourself*)*

1. ☐ People must love you or you will be miserable.

2. ☐ Making mistakes is terrible.

3. ☐ You are an awful human being—you're no good.

4. ☐ It is terrible when things go wrong.

5. ☐ Your emotions can't be controlled.

6. ☐ You should really be worried about threatening situations.

7. ☐ Self-discipline is *too* hard for you to achieve.

8. ☐ You must depend upon other people.

9. ☐ Your childhood must always affect you.

10. ☐ You just can't stand the way some people act.

11. ☐ Every problem has a perfect solution—so keep looking.

12. ☐ You should be better than others.

13. ☐ If others criticize you, you must have done something wrong.

14. ☐ You can't change what you think.

15. ☐ You should help everyone who needs it.

16. ☐ You must never show any weakness.

17. ☐ Healthy people don't get upset.

18. ☐ There is one true love.

19. ☐ You should never hurt anyone.

20. ☐ There is a magic cure for your problems.

21. ☐ It's someone else's responsibility to solve your problems.

22. ☐ Strong people don't ask for help.

23. ☐ You can do things *only* when you're in the mood—when you feel up to it.

24. ☐ Possible is the same as probable—if something bad can happen to you, it probably will.

25. ☐ You are inferior.

26. ☐ You are always in the spotlight—people watch you.

27. ☐ People ought to do what you want them to.

28. ☐ Giving up is the best policy.

29. ☐ Change is awful.

30. ☐ Knowing how your problems started when you were young is essential.

31. ☐ Everybody should trust you.

32. ☐ If you are not happy, something is wrong with you.

33. ☐ There is a secret, terrible part of you that controls your life.

34. ☐ Working on your problems is too scary.

35. ☐ The world ought to be fair.

36. ☐ You are not responsible for what you do sometimes.

37. ☐ Anxiety is always dangerous.

38. ☐ You should be able to control another person's behavior.

39. ☐ If you just had enough willpower, you wouldn't have these problems.

40. ☐ You must always make the right decision.

Now count up the number of statements that you did *not* check. If this number is greater than ten, I want you to go back over those that you did not check (otherwise continue to the next paragraph). Go back over each of the nonchecked statements again and ask yourself, "Has the Voice ever said this to me under any circumstance, at any time, in any place?" You may want to check some of those that you left blank. When you finish, continue to the next paragraph.

Now I want you to notice something interesting about these forty Voice messages—the ones you checked and the ones you did not check. Each one of them has something in common with the others. There is a single thread that binds all of them together, and this single thread is a clue, a very critical clue to an important attribute of the Voice. The one thing that all of these statements have in common is that *they are lies.* They are distortions of reality. They are flawed statements. One of the very first things I want you to learn about the Voice, and one of the things I never, ever want you to forget is, THE VOICE ALWAYS LIES.

When I say that the Voice always lies I mean that every time the Voice talks to you it is distorting a portion of reality. It is this distortion that causes the pain in your life.

Listening to the Voice, then, is not merely hearing its words, but also understanding how its message is flawed. You will be perfecting your ability to do this in chapter six, and eventually you will be able to quickly find the flaw in everything the Voice says. To start you along that road, I want you to find the flaw in each one of the forty common Voice messages. In your notebook, number a page from one to forty. Then re-phrase each Voice message so as to make it better match reality. When you have finished all forty messages, you will find answers at the end of the chapter.

As you go through each message, you will quickly become aware that one of the ways the Voice distorts reality is with the use of extreme language. As your eye moves down the list you will notice that many messages use words that express extreme ideas. Words like "always," "never," "should," "must," and "ought" are common examples of trick words the Voice uses to make you powerless. Not all of the flaws will have an easily identifiable extreme word. Sometimes the flaw will be conceptual. Nevertheless, there is always a flaw in everything the Voice says. When you have completed this assignment, go on to begin your Voice Diary.

Voice Diary

To become proficient at fighting the Voice, you must slow it down. Slowing it down is similar to learning any new skill in slow motion. For instance, if you are learning a new dance step, it helps to walk through the motions slowly and then gradually speed up the dance as you become more familiar with the steps. Slowing down the Voice can be done in two ways: verbal and written.

Verbal awareness can be accomplished by repeating out loud (when no one is present!) exactly what the Voice is saying to you. Don't worry if you cannot identify everything it says. The fact that you are attending and slowing it down verbally will eventually help you to identify all that the Voice says to you. Although at first you may feel silly talking aloud when you are alone, you will find that carrying on a verbal conversation with the Voice is a powerful method of tuning in to its destructive messages.

Another way of slowing down the Voice even further is to write down everything it says. This can be done by expanding your Emotions Diary to four columns. The information you need consists of (1) the time of day, (2) the situation, (3) the destructive emotions you are feeling, and (4) what the Voice is saying to you. Each column in the Voice Diary is labelled: Time, Situation, Voice. Look at the sample Voice Diary below to get an idea of what you need to do.

Time	Situation	Voice
9:00 A.M.	Slept in late	Your stupid husband forgot to wake you up.
Noon	Friend coming for lunch	You can't stand being trapped in your own house—as long as she is here, you won't be able to eat what you want.
3:00 P.M.	Pick up kids from school	You should not have been late getting your kids from school.
3:30 P.M.	Watching soaps	You are really a bad mother—a totally worthless human being.
8:00 P.M.	Reading paper	What if you are late again and someone kidnaps your children? You wouldn't be able to handle a tragedy like that.
8:15 P.M.	Reading paper	Do you feel all that anxiety right now? It feels like its going to get out of control. It's getting worse!

To do an effective job of keeping a Voice Diary you will probably have to keep it for at least a week before proceeding to the next chapter. Again, you will more than likely have to keep notes in a small notebook during the day and transfer this information to your Voice Diary each evening.

As you write down all of this information, you need to identify the facts of the situation. This data will help you to objectively discover what is actually happening rather than what the Voice says is happening. When you know what the Voice is saying to you, you will be in a better position to learn the technique of Voice Fighting. Voice Fighting is like a competitive event in which a person gains an advantage by knowing as much as possible about the opponent. This is, of course, why professional sports teams spend so many tiresome hours viewing videotapes of their opponent's behavior. At this point, knowledge is power!

Remember the following points as you keep your Voice Diary this week:

1. *All* of your destructive emotions are caused by habitual, destructive thinking patterns.

2. These destructive, negative thoughts belong to the Voice, not to you.

3. It is imperative that you learn to listen to the Voice and hear everything it is telling you.

4. Since the Voice is so quick, you need to slow it down. Repeat out loud what it says to you and write down what it says in your Voice Diary.

5. Be sure to use the second person pronoun "you" in the third column. Pretend you are a journalist at an interview and are writing down everything the Voice says about you.

6. To be successful in your Voice Awareness, it is essential that you separate yourself from the Voice. Refuse to take ownership of any more negative thoughts.

As you become more familiar with your Voice, you will begin to notice patterns and commonalities between many of the messages. In their book, *Thoughts and Feelings*, McKay, Davis, and Fanning have provided a summary of distorted thinking that matches very closely the kind of flaws the Voice uses with you. Read the list below carefully (there is no need to memorize it) so that you will begin to recognize these flaws as you keep your Voice Diary. The authors of this list do not mention the Voice, but their summary is a perfect example of what the Voice tries to do to you.

15 Voice Flaw Categories

1. **Filtering.** The Voice takes negative details and magnifies them while filtering out all positive aspects of a situation.

2. **Polarized Thinking.** The Voice tells you that things are black and white, good or bad. You have to be perfect or you're a failure. There is no middle ground!

3. **Overgeneralization.** The Voice insists on a general conclusion based on a single incident or piece of evidence. If something bad happens once, you can expect it to happen over and over again.

4. **Mind Reading.** The Voice tells you what people are feeling and why they act the way they do. In particular, the Voice is able to divine what people are thinking about you.

5. **Catastrophizing.** The Voice convinces you a disaster is imminent. As soon as you hear about a problem, the Voice starts to list a series of "what if's." What if you lose control and get fat? What if you can't stop binging?

6. **Personalization.** The Voice has convinced you that everything others do or say is some kind of reaction to you. It constantly compares you to those around you, trying to convince you that they are smarter, better looking, and so on.

7. **Control Fallacies.** Since the Voice controls your life, you see yourself as helpless, a victim of fate. On the other hand, it has you convinced that you are responsible for the pain or happiness of everyone around you.

8. **Fallacy of Fairness.** The Voice makes you feel resentful because you think you know what's fair but other people won't agree with you.

9. **Blaming.** The Voice either gets you to hold other people responsible for your pain or to blame yourself for every conceivable problem in your life.

10. **Shoulds.** The Voice has given you a list of ironclad rules about how you and other people should act. People who break the rules make you resentful, and you feel guilty if you violate the rules.

11. **Emotional Reasoning.** The Voice has convinced you that what you feel must be true—automatically. If you *feel* fat, then you must *be* fat.

12. **Fallacy of Change.** The Voice lies by telling you that other people will change to suit you if you must pressure or cajole them enough. Of course, the reason you need to change other people is because your happiness depends entirely on their behavior.

13. **Global Labeling.** The Voice generalizes one or two qualities into a negative global judgment. "Since you don't do well in math, that proves you're stupid."

14. **Being Right.** The Voice continually has you on trial to prove that your opinions and actions are correct. Being wrong is unthinkable, and the Voice has you going to any length to demonstrate your rightness.

15. **Heaven's Reward Fallacy.** Once again, the Voice has you believing that all your sacrifice and self-denial will pay, as if there were some-

one keeping score. Of course, the Voice is merely setting you up because you feel bitter when the reward doesn't come.

Be sure you feel comfortable about your ability to hear the Voice before continuing on to the next chapter. It is also important to understand that the Voice *always* lies and to be able to find the flaw in its messages. You may also want to read this chapter over several times while you spend about a week working on your diary.

Answers for the Common Voice Message Flaws

1. People must love you or you will be miserable.

The truth of the matter is that nobody *has* to love you—not even your own mother. It would be nice if everybody did love you, but there are no guarantees that anybody will. *Must* is an absolute word which puts pressure on you to be perfect and to feel guilty if you're not. The Voice is telling you that you *must* do everything in your power to get people to love you or you will be a miserable person. This is unrealistic and you could never hope to achieve this impossible goal.

If someone special doesn't love you, you will not be miserable. You may feel hurt, angry, or frustrated but miserable is one of those "awfulizer" words that make everything much worse than it really is.

2. Making mistakes is terrible.

The word "terrible" is a complete exaggeration. Making mistakes is inconvenient and human! You cannot learn from them if you think they are catastrophic. You only sink more deeply and spin your wheels trying to be "more perfect."

3. You are an awful human being.

Another totally unrealistic statement by the Voice. You are *not* an awful human being. You are the sum total of all your life experiences. Though you may think you've done some pretty awful things, these things are not what you *are*. This is a judgmental statement indicating that people are either good or bad.

4. It is terrible when things go wrong.

You may feel uncomfortable or anxious when things do not go as planned. But it is *not* "terrible." Life has lots of unpredictability. That's what makes it so fascinating. The word "terrible" again sets up a state of panic in your mind—just what the Voice wants. The minute you start feeling how "terrible" everything is, you start feeling hopeless. The Voice likes hopelessness.

5. Your emotions cannot be controlled.

This is untrue, as you will find out in this book. "Can't" expresses help-lessness. You *can* control your emotions by controlling the Voice. The Voice is what triggers your destructive emotions.

6. You should really be worried about threatening situations.

The words "you should" reveal a strong outside influence dictating and judging your actions. That strong outside influence is the Voice. You can be concerned, but you don't have to be worried. You can tell the Voice that worrying accomplishes nothing. Threatening situations are uncom-fortable but worrying about them only makes them worse.

7. Self-discipline is too hard for you to achieve.

"Too" is the key word here. Self-discipline can be very difficult at times, but it is not impossible to achieve. It takes perseverance and lots of repeti-tive, hard work. The Voice is just trying to set you up for another failure so you'll not even begin your personal improvement program.

8. You must depend on other people.

There's that word "must" again, putting pressure on you to give up your independent thinking by always depending on others for what is "right," "wrong," "good," or "bad." Listen to yourself and learn to depend on yourself. The Voice wants you to think you are helpless and can't do any-thing for yourself. You have intelligence and a good mind.

This statement is also an exaggeration in that it says, in effect, you must depend on others completely. True, you may need to lean on others now and then by asking their opinions. However, your decisions ultimate-ly depend on you.

9. Your childhood must always affect you.
Pure nonsense! Yes, your childhood has much to do with who you are now, but it need not affect the way you run your life in the here-and-now. You can transcend your childhood. The first step is to recognize some of the things that happened in your childhood, forgive your parents and yourself for being less than perfect, and then go on with your life. Forgiveness is the key, I think.

10. You just can't stand the way some people act.

Another exaggeration! Some of the things that people do and say will annoy you. The Voice, however, is trying to tell you these people are the sum total of all their faults and annoying ways. The Voice is asking you to expect perfection from other fallible human beings.

You may think, sometimes, that you can't stand the way you act and perhaps respond negatively when others act in a way you find imperfect. Seeing others as fearful, instead of as "attacking" you, will help you to treat them with gentleness and understanding.

11. Every problem has a perfect solution.

There is no such thing as the "perfect solution." If you expect to wait and wait until you eventually find the perfect solution, you will take forever to solve the problem at hand. There is no pot of gold at the end of the rainbow. You will also set yourself up for failure by expecting to find the perfect solution.

12. You should be better than others.

There's that strong outside influence again (the Voice)—the one that dictates to you and judges you. Why should you be better than others? Because the Voice tells you that you should be? Ridiculous! This statement is unreasonable. You don't expect others to be better than you, do you? The Voice is asking you to constantly compare yourself to other people. Just be yourself and let others be themselves.

13. If others criticize you, you must have done something wrong.

You certainly have believed this one for a long time. This statement is similar to "If you do things that are bad, you *are* bad." Another total lie. Remember, others may find fault with you for reasons stemming from their own insecurities. Also, the word "wrong" is needlessly judgmental.

14. You can't change what you think.

This is the only thing you really *can* change, so the statement is a complete untruth. The Voice is just trying to keep you locked up in your misery. Remember, "can't" denotes helplessness. Say instead, "I *want* to change what I think, even though it will require lots of work." This makes the task a very real possibility.

15. You should help everyone who needs it.

The Voice is saying you are responsible for the needs of everyone around you. You can't please all of the people all of the time. You can't be all things to all people. It is good to be helpful and to be thoughtful, but not at the expense of forgetting to take care of yourself. Besides, you don't have the capacity to help everyone, and people have to *want* to help themselves. The Voice is trying to make you feel guilty if you fail at helping everyone. Just do the best you can.

16. You must never show any weakness.

This statement is loaded with untruths, even though you've believed it all your life. "You must" denotes that you absolutely *have to* be perfect no matter what. "You must" never gives you any room at all for error. "You must never show any" says that *all* weakness is bad.

Weakness is a very human and compassionate quality. Strong people are often the only people who are capable of admitting they have any weaknesses. You need to have weakness in order to have strength.

17. Healthy people don't get upset.

You've thought that if you were only healthy, slender, and therefore perfect, you would automatically become serene and calm. The truth is, healthy people allow themselves to get upset from time to time. They know there is nothing wrong with it, that it will not lead to insanity. They have effective ways of dealing with turmoil and are able to feed themselves constructive thoughts which then generate constructive emotions. Getting upset is not *bad*.

18. There is one true love.

I guess most people really *do* want to believe this. You may not like the fact that it isn't true, because you want it to be true. The truth is that love is a *human* emotion and therefore fallible. Besides, one person isn't capable of fulfilling all the needs of another person. This myth places extra, unnecessary pressure on the one being loved. He or she must never fail being the "true love" whom you have labelled. In the same regard, don't think that you need to be a perfect, true lover, either. It just isn't possible. You can love any number of people in your life, but making the relationship succeed is a matter of commitment and hard work. It isn't a matter of finding the "perfect" mate.

19. You should never hurt anyone.

Those wonderful words "should" and "never" again. They certainly don't leave any room for doubt, do they? Not hurting people is good in theory, but people *will* get hurt—even if you do not mean to hurt them. Sometimes when you stand up for yourself and are truthful about your feelings, another person might view it as rejection and feel hurt. Remember, though, people have to *allow* themselves to be hurt.

20. There is a magic cure for your problems.

The Voice is trying to get you to believe that one morning you are going to wake up and find you are cured of all problems and perfectly in control. Obviously, this won't happen. You just need to work on your problems every day and face them realistically.

21. It's someone else's responsibility to solve your problems.

The Voice wants you to think you are incapable of solving your own problems, that you are helpless and *must* have someone else do all the work and give you the answers. But really it is your responsibility. You can ask for guidance and for suggestions from others, but ultimately, you have to make the commitment to change.

22. *Strong people don't ask for help.*

Another variation of "It's weak and therefore *bad* to need help." The truth is, strong people ask for help when they need it because they know there is no shame in needing help. Actually, the stronger you are, the more likely you are to ask for help. You know both your strengths and your weaknesses and accept yourself as being human. The Voice is telling you another wearisome untruth.

23. *You can do things only when you're in the mood.*

This one is very familiar. You may think that if you put something off because you're not in the mood, the time will come when you *are* in the mood to do it. Another variation is, "You can relax *only* when you're in the mood to relax." The opposite is true. You need to learn how to relax when you're *not* in the mood. The Voice is giving you excuses for your avoidance of responsibility to yourself.

24. *Possible is the same as probable.*

"It is possible that my guests will think I'm a terrible housekeeper" translates into "My guests *will* think I'm a terrible housekeeper." This is a typical worry statement. Most things you worry about never happen.

25. *You are inferior.*

Of course you are not inferior! You may *think* at times that you are inferior, but that is because you are listening to the Voice without evaluating what it is saying to you. You have a right to your lifestyle and your choices in life. Because you make mistakes doesn't make you inferior. You are no better or no worse than the next person. The Voice wants you to feel subservient and victimized by the demands of others. The irony here is that the Voice is telling you that you are inferior in one ear while telling you that you must be better than others (message 12) in the other ear.

26. *You are always in the spotlight.*

Or: everyone is watching you *all* the time, so you'd better not screw up. The truth is, people are usually too concerned about themselves and their own problems to be watching you all the time.

27. *People ought to do what you want them to.*

The Voice is telling you that your wishes are more important than those of other people. Everyone's needs are personal and equal. By wishing correct behavior from other people, you automatically judge what they are doing. You don't want them judging you, do you? Besides, you can't wish people into doing anything. Live and let live.

28. *Giving up is the best policy.*

The Voice loves this one. It's so easy to throw up your hands and say, "I can't. I quit." When you do this, you give the Voice complete dominance over your life. When you give up, the Voice has the perfect opportunity to feed you all kinds of destructive messages. Instead of quitting, work harder at feeding yourself constructive thoughts.

29. Change is awful.

Change can be painful because the consequences are often unknown, but it is not *awful*. Change can give you new opportunities to grow and learn. Change keeps your mind open and your life from becoming stagnant.

30. Knowing how your problems started when you were young is essential.

It's good to have perspective and to find out what started you on your roller coaster ride into destructive behavior, but it is not essential. What is essential is that you start *now* by changing how you think. Besides, you can't change what happened when you were young. Everyone around you probably did the best they could with what information they had at the time. You probably did the best you could do. Remember: forgive yourself and others.

31. Everybody should trust you.

Trust is something that is earned and cannot be considered a "should." People often have their own built-in mistrust. Don't let that bother you. Just concentrate on being trustworthy to yourself and the rest will come in time if you are patient. Be true to yourself.

32. If you are not happy, something is wrong with you.

This just isn't possible for any human being. The Voice is trying to make you feel guilty if you aren't "Little Miss Sunny Skies" every day of your life. You'll always have your down days. This is just part of life. Without some sadness, there certainly wouldn't be any happiness. Being a "full" human being involves both.

33. There is a secret, terrible part of you that controls your life.

The Voice wants you to think you are a slave to some kind of "evil" force within you. The truth of the matter is this "secret" thing within has been the Voice all along and you just didn't know it. You have been a slave to the destructive emotions the Voice has been giving you. You have forgotten to look for the "good" qualities you possess. There is no terrible part of you. I know you've thought that for a long time, but it's just the Voice trying to stop you from believing that *you* are in control of *your* life.

34. Working on your problems is scary.

For you, diving into the deep murky waters of the past might be scary. But, working on your problems in the present is not scary at all. The work is very rewarding, especially when you begin to see results. Working on your problems is a challenge. By saying that "working on your problems is scary," the Voice wants you to be overwhelmed by all the obstacles in your path to recovery.

35. The world ought to be fair.

Maybe it *ought* to be, but it isn't! That's just a fact of life. Remember, you cannot change the world you live in or the people in it. But you can change how you perceive the world, how you perceive others, and how you perceive yourself.

36. You are not responsible for what you do sometimes.

As a thinking adult with the power of choice, you are responsible for your behavior. The Voice wants you to remain a child forever—blaming everyone and everything except yourself for the way you act. Condemning yourself, however, is worthless because it robs you of the energy you need to take positive action. You are not responsible for another person's feelings, either—just for your own actions and behavior toward others. If you have behaved in such a way as to violate someone's rights, the only remedy is action on your part. You can rectify the situation by offering an apology and doing something to make restitution.

37. Anxiety is always dangerous.

Anxiety cannot hurt you. Anxiety is nothing more than an exaggerated physical reaction related to normal feelings. You can tolerate moderate anxiety by realizing that performance anxiety will *improve* your ability to handle any situation. Extreme anxiety can be very stressful but this stress can be reduced by doing your stress reduction exercises such as natural breathing, deep muscle relaxation, and mental imagery. You also need to realize the Voice is trying to make everything much worse than it really is. Not only does moderate anxiety not hurt you, it gives you the warning signal to let go of the stress which has been building up in your life.

38. You should be able to control another person's behavior.

The Voice is giving you another guilty "should." You can't do anything about another person's behavior—only about your own. You are also not responsible for other people's behavior. If you see that someone is upset or thoughtful about something, you may automatically assume that you must have done something to make that person upset or that you could have in some way prevented him or her from being upset. Once again, live and let live.

39. Willpower alone can solve your problems.

"If you just had enough willpower. . ." How many times has the Voice said that to you? Well, the Voice knows that you, like most people, are a little short on willpower. If it can get you to believe willpower is your missing ingredient to a better life, it will lead you into a blind alley. Problems will come up whether or not you have willpower. Not willpower, but changing your thoughts from destructive to constructive can help you to solve your problems. Don't strive for willpower, because you will fall short—it's too close to the perfection ideal.

40. You must always make the the right decision.

If you always made the right decision, nothing would be challenging anymore. We're here on this earth to learn from our mistakes. Also, there are no "right" and "wrong" decisions. These are judgmental words the Voice uses to make you feel guilty. Sometimes what may seem like the "wrong" decision at the time will turn out just the opposite and surprise you. You can only make the best decision possible at the time with whatever resources you have. Don't condemn yourself for not being perfect.

Homework

1. The major goal of this chapter is to learn what the Voice sounds like. Remember that *speed* and *secrecy* will make this difficult. You will be slowing down what the Voice says to you by writing in your Voice Diary.

The secrecy weapon is best combatted by watching your pronouns. Most people have an internal dialogue that goes something like this: "I am so stupid and dumb. I can't do anything right. No, you're not. You don't make any more mistakes than the average person."

These pronouns are backward—the "I" is related to negative thoughts, the "you" is related to positive thoughts. You must reverse this process and use the pronoun "you" when the Voice is talking and "I" when you are thinking positively. As you fill in your diary, pretend you are a newspaper reporter and writing down what someone (the Voice) is saying to you.

By watching your pronouns, you will avoid owning the negative thoughts and will give them to the Voice, where they belong. When my clients call me back months after therapy has ended to tell me that they are having a setback, 99 percent of the time they are reversing their pronouns. Watching your pronouns will help you clarify the mental confusion which the Voice loves to create.

2. It is time for you to begin adding a noisy environment to your progressive relaxation. Eventually, you will want to be able to relax regardless of what the noise level is around you. You can begin by gradually going from quiet to loud noise. Use a radio and tune to a station that you absolutely detest—or to a program that is very distracting, like a talk show. Turn the volume down as far as possible. You want to know that it is

there, but you do not want it to bother you. As time goes on, you can begin to turn the volume up little by little. If you do this systematically, you will be able to relax even when it is very noisy.

3. If you have not already done so, find the flaws in each of the 40 common Voice messages. You may find different flaws than the ones I have given you in this chapter. That is okay. The important thing to learn is that every time the Voice talks to you, it is lying to you. It does this by distorting reality, but does so in such a way that you think its messages are quite reasonable.

Skills Checklist

- ☐ Morning rituals (2)
- ☐ Evening rituals (2)
- ☐ Relaxation (7 muscle groups) with noise
- ☐ Identify your common Voice messages
- ☐ Find the flaws in common Voice messages
- ☐ Become familiar with the 15 Voice flaws
- ☐ Voice Diary

5

Getting in Touch With
Your Feelings

The advantage of the emotions is that they lead us astray

–OSCAR WILDE, 1891

As a member of the human race, you are an emotional being, like it or not. You respond to life, people, and circumstances with feelings. One of the means the Voice will use against you is emotional confusion. Almost all Deadly Dieters have emotional mood swings that are totally beyond their personal control. Many times there are so many emotions taking place that it feels like you are drowning in a sea of feelings. The Voice will use these experiences of yours to your disadvantage. It does this in two different ways.

The first is to make it difficult for you to identify and pinpoint your emotions accurately. If you were to have several stressful encounters at work, you might later describe your day as "rotten." Or you might tell someone you were "not feeling good." You might even describe yourself as being "bummed out" or some equally vague phrase. The problem with these emotional descriptions is that they are *global* and *nonspecific*. Because the Voice has gotten you to "generalize" about the problem, you're left with a sense of confusion—a "what can I do?" feeling.

A second way that the Voice will confuse you is to get you to trust your emotions when it comes to decision making. Many people treat feelings as factual information. You have probably heard people say, "I really don't know why I want to do that, it's just a feeling I have."

These two Voice tricks—an inability to zero in on your emotions and a tendency to make decisions based on how you feel—can contribute greatly to becoming lost in the Control Cycle and allowing the Voice to continue running your life. For this reason it is important to learn how to bring the anarchy of your emotional life under your personal control.

To begin, you must learn to see how your emotions are related to the rest of your experiences. Most people believe that emotions are caused by what happens in their environment.

For instance, if you were asked by someone why you were feeling angry or depressed, you would probably identify the source of your emotion as some person or event outside of yourself. You might say that you were depressed because something bad had happened to you. Or you might report that an unkind remark had made you feel angry.

These feelings, in turn, can act as strong influences on your behavior. You may feel justified in being curt or sarcastic because someone "made you angry." You may retreat into silence because you felt hurt. You may punish yourself because of a guilty feeling that you've done wrong. You may avoid things that "make you afraid."

The conventional wisdom is that *events cause emotions*, emotions generate a *behavioral response*, and the behavior in turn results in certain *consequences*. This chain can be illustrated in the following diagram as a four-link experience chain.

Events → Emotions → Behavior → Consequences

Although this sequence appears perfectly reasonable, it has a major flaw in it, related to the issue of personal control. But to what extent can you control each of the links in this chain? When you look at the first link, it is apparent that this area of your experience is generally beyond your immediate control. Most of us recognize the fact that we have very little control over external events such as the weather, other people's behavior, and the working of machines. You can fine tune your car until it runs like a Swiss watch, and it can still break down in the middle of a country road on a dark night. You can choose a person who is honest, loyal, and considerate for a friend, and he can still disappoint you when you least expect it. Let's face it: we have very little control over what happens to us.

The second link, feelings, also seems beyond control. If you have ever been depressed and tried to feel better by telling yourself, "I'm going to feel happy now," you know how futile this kind of effort can be. And the stronger the emotion is, the more difficult it is to change. Emotions like irrational fear, resentment, guilt, and depression seem to have a life of their own—it seems like you have to just hang on till the storm blows itself out.

Likewise, everyone knows how difficult it can be to control a habitual response. The response seems ingrained, almost automatic. It can take mountains of willpower to keep your voice low when feeling angry, or to keep from becoming lethargic when you're depressed, or to stop yourself from avoiding things that make you extremely anxious.

There you have it! You wind up with the disheartening discovery that all the links in your experience chain are essentially beyond your control. If this experience chain were an accurate depiction of reality, we could stop questioning it right now.

Fortunately, this common sense sequence of events—environment-feelings-behavior-consequences—has a vital link missing: the "think link." The following sequence is more representative of the way things really are.

Events → Thoughts → Emotions → Behavior → Consequences

Notice that between the event and your feelings are your thoughts. The truth is that *your thoughts are the cause of your feelings*. It is not what happens to you that makes you feel a certain way, but rather how you interpret what happens to you, the meaning you attach to the event. The same event may bring on very different feelings, depending on what you think. This is where the Voice can disrupt your entire life. If you let the Voice control your thinking, you will surely experience out-of-control emotions that overwhelm you.

Once you realize that your thoughts are at the base of all your emotions, you can begin to learn how to sort out your thoughts from your emotions. Although it is critically important that at any given moment you can distinguish between what you are thinking and what you are feeling, making this distinction is not always an easy task. One reason is that your feelings tend to be more intense than your thoughts. Even though both occur simultaneously, your feelings can be so overpowering that no amount of concentration can help you to identify your thinking. Trying to sort out your low-level thoughts from your high-level feelings is like trying to read a book while sitting on a red hot griddle. And while you are concentrating on your painful emotions, the Voice continues eating away at you without your knowledge.

The multiple meanings of the word "feel" can also make it difficult to sort out feelings and thoughts. We usually use the word to describe three different experiences. The most obvious is to describe an emotion: "I feel happy." We also use the word to describe sensations: "I feel tired." The most subtle and potentially confusing use of the word is to describe our thoughts, beliefs, and attitudes: "I feel that exercise is good for me." This is not a statement about your emotions, but rather an opinion about exercise.

You are most accurate in talking about your emotions when you use the form, "I feel _____," with an emotion word such as happy, frustrated, angry, or anxious in the blank. "I feel that you're always late" is a *judgment*, not an emotion. The phrase ' 'I feel that" usually indicates a thought, not a feeling. Similarly confused phrases are "I feel that the economy is going to the dogs" (an opinion) and "I feel that I have the right to act the way I want to" (an attitude).

Your thoughts are best expressed when you use the form, "I think or believe that _____." Any belief, attitude, or opinion can be put in this blank. When you find yourself using the phrase "I feel that," change it to "I think" or "I believe." The long-term benefit is that you will become able to quickly find out what the Voice is saying to you.

In addition to using feeling words when referring to thoughts, you may also use the word "feel" to tell people what is happening to your body. "I feel a pain in my left side" is a statement about your physiology, not your emotions. Unfortunately, we really have no better substitute for describing our bodily sensations than the word "feel." Even though you can "feel" tired, hungry, dizzy, or vibrant, you must remember that these are sensations, not emotions.

Exercise

For this exercise, you may find it helpful to be in a place where you feel comfortable. Choose a place where you can minimize distractions. When you are ready, spend a few minutes using your Natural Breathing to calm down. Then write the following phrase at the top of a piece of paper: "Now I see . . . "

Take five minutes to observe your environment and write down what you see around you. Then start another page. At the top of this page write the words, "Now I think . . . "

Again, after five minutes of identifying your thoughts, title another page, "Now I feel . . . " Be sure that you identify emotions on this page and not thoughts or sensations.

Constructive vs. Destructive Emotions

The Experience Chain shows that many of your intense feelings come about because of the way you interpret and think about specific events in your environment. Depending on the meaning you attach to it, the same event can trigger off very different thoughts. This can be illustrated by looking at the two branches of the Experience Chain below.

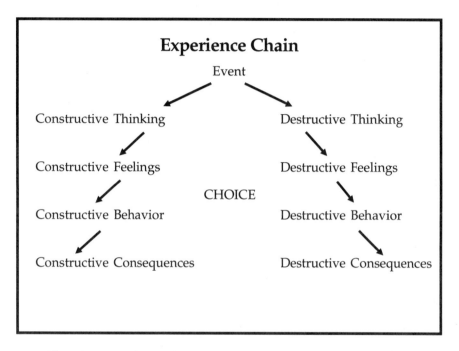

This diagram shows that any event can trigger off either destructive thinking—the Voice—or constructive thinking—you. If you go down the path of destructive thinking, you will then experience destructive feelings, followed by destructive behavior and negative consequences. But you can learn to think constructively after a triggering event, then you will experience constructive feelings, constructive behavior, and more positive consequences.

Your task, then, is threefold: (1) to become more aware of the Voice, (2) to get rid of the Voice, and (3) to replace it with more constructive thinking. The problem in reaching this goal is awareness. How can you listen to the Voice when some events are such strong triggers that you jump from the event to the destructive emotion in the blink of an eye? The transition can pass so quickly that you are not even aware of your Voice. In certain situations, you have probably even said to yourself, "I feel so guilty all of a sudden, for no reason at all." This feeling which seems to come "out of the blue," is still caused by the Voice, whether or not you are aware of it.

The solution to becoming aware of the lightening-like action of the Voice is to use your feelings and behavior as clues to what the Voice is saying to you. This coming-in-the-back-door approach uses your destructive feelings as a data base to uncover the Voice's secrecy weapon. When you feel angry, for example, you can trace the feeling back to the thoughts that precipitated it. Any emotion can be a red flag to go back and examine the thoughts, memories, and images immediately preceding it.

Types of Emotions

Unfortunately, most people with Deadly Diets have a rather foggy notion of what they are feeling at any given moment. You probably sort your feelings into two categories: pleasant or unpleasant. When you are having a bad day you may say something like, "I'm having a bad day," or "I'm feeling rotten today," or "Things are really going terrible."

These statements are much too vague to be of any practical use. It would be much better if you could be more specific when describing how you feel at any point in time. This can be done if you know that all of your unpleasant emotions can be further subdivided into two categories: constructive and destructive. That's right—some painful emotions are constructive. In fact, you will learn that most painful emotions are constructive. This means that there are three types of emotions: pleasant, unpleasant-destructive, and unpleasant-constructive. By learning the differences between these three categories, you can gain more control over your life.

The inability to tell the difference between destructive and constructive emotions is what causes such emotional confusion in Deadly Dieters. There are three good reasons for you to learn to separate these two types of unpleasant emotions: time, personal growth, and coping behaviors.

Time. Destructive and constructive emotions have differing influences on your time. Destructive emotions are protracted and lengthy. They just roll on and on, with no end in sight. Guilty, fearful, or depressed people tend to stay in their painful ruts for years. Constructive emotions, on the other hand, are time-limited. They run their course and inflict pain over a much shorter and limited time span. A police officer is plainly justified in feeling a surge of fear if caught in a shoot-out with a dangerous criminal. Unlike irrational fear, however, rational fear subsides within minutes or hours after the real trigger is removed. The phrase "time heals all wounds" readily applies to constructive emotions. They really do tend to subside with the passage of time.

Personal growth. Destructive emotions are like cancers. They eat away at you, destroy you, and ruin your life. Depression or unreasonable fear can tear you apart if left unchecked. This does not mean that a panic attack or a strong bout of depression can physically hurt you. The feelings by themselves cannot damage you, and with the skills you will be learning you will soon have control over them. But in the long run, destructive emotions can disrupt your life if you don't learn to change them. They turn your emotional life into a wasteland. On the other hand, constructive emotions build you up and make you stronger. Boredom, frustration, or anger energizes you and makes you a more solid, more productive person in the process. It is when these constructive emotions, such as boredom, are overwhelmed by one of the destructive emotions, such as helplessness, that you begin to bog down.

If you have ever known someone who has gone through a lot of pain and suffering, you know what I am talking about. When you listen to this person after the painful event is finished, you notice that the person is more mature and has more depth of character, tolerance, and other virtues that we humans value.

On the other hand, if you have ever known a person who has been born with that proverbial "silver spoon in his mouth," you are likely to see the opposite effect. The person who has never had anything go wrong or who has easily reached personal goals and has never had to struggle with life's difficulties can often be described as quite shallow. It takes no more than a few minutes of conversation to realize how empty such a person is.

Unpleasant-constructive emotions are a necessary evil in an imperfect world. They have value because they often build character and teach basic and necessary truths about life and humanity in general. They encourage personal growth, while destructive emotions inhibit personal growth.

Coping behaviors. Destructive emotions can be power-zapping. They leave you de-energized, lifeless, with little incentive to do anything. Or else they force you to do something totally counterproductive, which makes your situation even worse. The bulimic person who feels guilty over a binge will often keep right on binging, rather than keeping to her strategy for success. Likewise, depression never energized anybody to do anything. It leaves you stuck. Constructive emotions, on the other hand, energize you by getting you to do something that betters your situation. They get you moving to take corrective action. A constructive alternative to guilt, for example, is remorse. A husband who belligerently downgrades his wife has good reason to feel regret, and this feeling may motivate him to resolve the situation (make amends, apologize, change his behavior, and so on). If he chooses to wallow in personal guilt, however, he will probably not take any positive action, but instead continue to feel guilty and perpetuate his unwarranted behavior.

Six Destructive Emotions

Our work at the clinic has led to the discovery of six—and only six— destructive emotions at the heart of all Deadly Diets. If you can learn how to control these six destructive emotions, rather than being controlled by them, significant progress can be made in your personal life.

Depression

Depression is something almost everyone at some time or other has experienced. Yet, while most people have only had to deal with it temporarily, Deadly Dieters usually experience chronic depression. In fact, depression is so common that it is often misdiagnosed by mental health professionals who have had little or no experience with Deadly Diets.

Chronic depression is destructive because it usually lasts for a very long time. Seldom does it get better with time, even though improvement is possible. While you are experiencing depression, you are being destroyed emotionally. It is like an invisible cancer that eats away at you until only a shell of the real you remains. Depression also saps your energy so that you begin to cut back on activities that are part of your everday routine. The clue that you are depressed is the lethargy that surrounds your behavior.

The pleasant alternative to depression is what people dream of when they feel depressed: happiness, joy, and feeling good. The unpleasant-constructive counterpart of depression is sadness or grief. Depression is unnatural and inappropriate, while sadness is a very human, natural emotion. For instance, when a loved one dies, feeling depressed is destructive and unnecessary, as the depression in fact makes it more difficult to cope with the personal loss. However, it is natural to feel grief and sadness over the loss.

When you are depressed you engage in "lethargy" behaviors; when you are sad you cry. Not only do we intuitively know that crying makes us feel better, but also researchers at the University of Minnesota have discovered two important neurotransmitters (brain chemicals) in tears. This may imply that crying might be a chemical release for emotional stress. They have also found that the tears caused by eye irritation are chemically different from tears of sadness. Tears of sadness may have important consequences for our emotional well-being.

Subjectively and chemically, sadness and depression differ from one another. To see how these two emotions effect us differently, consider Adam: a depressed widower who has been without a job for five years because of his depression. When he says, "First I lost my job, then my wife died. That was five years ago. I've felt lifeless and gloomy ever since," he is describing the longevity of depression and its destructive effects on his life.

His friends often say that they want Adam to feel happy again—as we have already seen, this is the pleasant alternative to depression. But this emotion would be totally inappropriate for Adam's situation.

A constructive substitute for this depression would be some months of sadness and grief. This would be a normal, natural, constructive response to the death of a loved one. In his book, *A Severe Mercy*, Sheldon Vanauken describes the process of grief he forced himself through upon the death of his wife. He deliberately made himself look at old photographs and listen to their favorite music in order to feel the sadness and pain. In doing this he knew that he was engaging in a healing process brought on by the grief and tears.

This constructive emotion hurts—like all constructive-unpleasant emotions. But it does not leave you drained of all life and energy. Grief and sadness act as healing balms. Eventually you recover and become stronger.

To help you discover the difference between pleasant, unpleasant-constructive, and unpleasant-destructive emotions, complete the following worksheet. Identify those situations that make you feel happy, sad, and depressed.

HAPPY	DEPRESSED	SAD
_____	_____	_____
_____	_____	_____
_____	_____	_____
_____	_____	_____

Guilt

Feeling guilty is a waste of time. It stops you from taking positive action for yourself. It acts like quicksand. You feel stuck, and the more you struggle, the more you sink. As you wallow in your guilt, it becomes increasingly difficult to go on with any real program on self-improvement. You become incapable of making decisions that can improve the quality of your life.

Associated with your guilt is the frequent use of judgmental words like *should, ought, must,* and *have to.* The guilt brought on by the use of these words compels you to punish yourself. Many of these punishing directives can be so exacting and impossible to follow that you feel even more guilt for not following through. And if your own punishment is not severe enough, you can always find someone else to help you.

Many people think the pleasant opposite of guilt, a feeling of accomplishment or self-esteem, is the only alternative to guilt. This is not true. Instead of feeling guilty and punishing yourself, it would be more productive and constructive to feel remorse or regret. Because we are imperfect people and often hurt others, intentionally or otherwise, it is proper to feel regret for what we have done. The behavior associated with remorse is reconciliation. It is a corrective one in which you apologize for having done something to damage the other person or your relationship. You take action to make up for the wrong you have inflicted.

Let's listen to Betty expressing her guilt: "I feel so awful, so guilty. I just caved into my fears all this week. I know I shouldn't have. I blew it! I'll never get my act together." Betty has set up an unreasonable set of rules: never make mistakes and never give into fear. By trying to live with these impossible rules, she tends to live in a perpetual state of guilt. All that is really happening is the expression of fallible human nature. Everyone makes mistakes. Since her set of rules have come to her from outside and have been accepted without question as a necessary way of life, her sense of shame becomes overwhelming. This traps her into a cycle where even more rules are broken and more guilt experienced. The guilt keeps her moving in circles. Remorse would put her on a straight line toward taking corrective action. "I really regret having blown it this weekend. But I recognize that I am still on the road to recovery and have a long way to go. I am getting stronger, but I'm not strong enough to make it through the weekend yet. Someday, I will do it."

Remember, guilt results in self-punishment, while remorse and regret result in reconciliation. Since we cannot stop ourselves from ever hurting someone, we must accept regret as a fact of life. We live in a broken world, a world dominated by the hurts that people inflict on each other. Our task as human beings is not to pretend this doesn't happen or to wish for utopia. We must daily engage in the business of reconciliation, healing the broken lives and wounds that are a part of living together.

Complete another worksheet to help you identify the differences between self-esteem, guilt, and remorse.

SELF-ESTEEM   REMORSE   GUIDE

_____   _____   _____

_____   _____   _____

_____   _____   _____

_____   _____   _____

Helplessness

When you feel helpless, you have a sense of being trapped and unable to deal with the specific situation. Helplessness keeps you from even trying to cope with whatever is happening to you. Consequently, the behavior that is often associated with helplessness is escape behavior—running away. This running away from your problems makes the helplessness even worse the next time around.

The pleasant alternative to feeling helpless is feeling powerful and strong. The constructive alternative to helplessness is a feeling of weakness. After all, that is what we human beings are: weak, frail, and imperfect.

When you can avoid the extremes of seeing yourself as either perfect or pathetic, then you can begin to understand yourself more realistically. These extremes can trap you into feeling helpless if you are unable to act strong and powerful when things go wrong unexpectedly. Accepting yourself as you are is always a good first step toward self-improvement.

If the behavior of helplessness is escape, then the behavior of weakness is self-improvement. By recognizing your own weaknesses, you can put energy into improving your personal skills. In this way you will begin to notice that out of your weakness will grow strength. Out of your helplessness will only come hopelessness.

Helplessness can become a self-fulfilling prophesy. Cathy: "I have anorexia and I just feel so out of control with my eating habits. Everybody else is *so* strong and I'm such an emotional marshmallow. I can't stand these feelings." As long as Cathy is convinced that she is incapable of doing anything positive about her problem, then this emotion—helplessness—will perpetuate itself through the self-fulfilling prophecy. The conviction of helplessness and lack of positive action to make personal changes form a downward spiral that will keep Cathy from making any constructive changes in her life.

Complete another worksheet for the following emotions.

STRENGTH   HELPLESSNESS   WEAKNESS

_____   _____   _____

_____   _____   _____

_____   _____   _____

_____   _____   _____

Resentment

Resentment is another destructive emotion with many synonyms—hatred, bitterness, and hostility, among others. It is an emotion that can singlehandedly destroy any relationship. Its pleasant counterparts are compassion, love, acceptance, and kindness. Unfortunately, many people have been told that these are the only alternatives to feeling resentful. This message is unfortunate because it does not allow you to feel the full range of human emotions.

The constructive alternative to resentment is anger. Anger is constructive because it is necessary in personal relationships. If you take any two people in the world and put them in the same room, you will eventually have friction. If they stay together long enough, there will be conflict. Anger is the emotion that clearly identifies conflict. The problem is that most people don't know how to use anger to deal with conflict creatively.

This confusion between anger and resentment causes many people to denounce anger as a social or moral evil. Yet, when you recognize the difference between anger and resentment, it is much easier to accept anger as a potentially positive emotion. Anger can help you become more intimate and caring with another person if—and it is a big if—you learn how to deal with it. (For an excellent resource for learning how to do this, see *Messages*, by McKay, Davis, and Fanning.) It is difficult to be angry with someone or something you don't care about. And yet many people think that the absence of anger is the goal of relationships. Have you ever heard someone describe their marriage by saying, "We've been married for fifteen years and have never had a cross word with one another"? To many people, this situation is the ideal. Actually such a couple should be pitied, because this anger means that they have never been deeply involved in each other's life.

A person who feels resentment and bitterness will most likely engage in retaliatory and vengeful behavior. A resentful person spends a lot of time "getting even" with other people or society in general. Family feuds that continue for years and even generations are fueled by the emotion of resentment, not anger. Let's listen to Debbie and hear what resentment sounds like. "I work my tail off for the boss, and he doesn't appreciate me, the rat. If I had the guts, I'd tell that jerk to take a flying leap. He makes me so mad! I feel like I'm going to blow up."

It is apparent that Debbie is not only concerned with her boss's behavior—whatever it is—but that she also insists on spending time evaluating his worth as a human being. By thinking of him as a "rat" and a "jerk" she is forcing herself to experience a destructive emotion rather than anger, a more constructive emotion. As with all other destructive emotions, the resentment will probably fester and slowly destroy her.

On the other hand, the angry person deals with the behavior of other people by requesting that they change their behavior. They do not waste their time evaluating the worth of the other person. This demand-for-change can be constructive and helpful.

Let's see how Debbie would sound if she were to be angry instead of resentful. "I'm really angry when you assume that I will work overtime anytime you want me to and then ask me at the last minute. I am willing to put in some overtime, but I want you to give me at least forty-eight hours' notice. As a single parent it is difficult for me to find someone to care for my daughter without at least that much notice."

By getting angry, instead of resentful, and expressing it appropriately to her boss, Debbie will get over the anger fairly quickly and will go on with her life.

TOLERANCE	RESENTMENT	ANGER
_____	_____	_____
_____	_____	_____
_____	_____	_____
_____	_____	_____

Unhealthy Anxiety

Unhealthy anxiety can be a terrifying, destructive emotion. It results from the expectation that something awful is going to happen in the near future. This anticipated catastrophe can be very specific or quite vague. It can be real or imagined. Nevertheless, if the anxiety is strong enough, it will keep you from a specific activity or event.

The behavior which is associated with unhealthy anxiety is avoidance. This is different from the escape behavior of helplessness. Instead of getting out of a stressful and painful situation, you avoid getting into it altogether.

Anxiety is always an anticipatory emotion in that it is focused on the future. It is not concerned with what is happening now, but with what may happen tomorrow or even a few minutes from now. Once unhealthy anxiety becomes associated with something in the future, you will do anything to avoid confronting that situation, whether it is eating, gaining weight, or being with certain people.

While the pleasant alternative to unhealthy anxiety is peace, calm, tranquility, and serenity, the constructive opposite is healthy anxiety. Healthy anxiety is normal in many situations, so long as it does not incapacitate you. This kind of anxiety is often referred to as "performance anxiety." It occurs whenever a person is expected to act in front of people who are going to evaluate that performance. People who perform for others—musicians, actors, and athletes—will tell you that performance anxiety is part of their job. In fact, many of these people will admit that if they are *not* experiencing anxiety just prior to performing, it often dulls their performance by taking them off the cutting edge so necessary to doing an outstanding job.

While unhealthy anxiety will incapacitate you, healthy anxiety will energize and motivate you to reach your personal goals. That is why it is important when sorting through personal feelings to be able to distinguish between healthy (constructive) and unhealthy (destructive) labels of anxiety. If you misinterpret healthy anxiety as something worse than it really is, you are likely to convert healthy anxiety to unhealthy anxiety.

Eve describes her unhealthy anxiety: "Oh, my gosh. I have to go to dinner with my friends this evening. What if I lose control and eat too much? Everybody will see what is happening and think I am such a fool. Not only will I make a fool of myself, but I will eat so much food that I will get fat and blow up like a blimp. That will be the ultimate tragedy."

Eve's example is one that every anoretic will find familiar. The "what ifs" are an essential part of the anoretic's destructive thinking patterns. And, of course, the anticipation of something awful happening is almost always worse than the actual event. One thing must be remembered—a person who has never experienced unhealthy anxiety has a difficult time trying to understand why it is so awful. Because of this, the anoretic who feels unhealthy anxiety often feels quite alone and misunderstood, unable to share this tremendous anxiety and its effects on her life.

TRANQUILITY	UNHEALTHY ANXIETY	HEALTHY ANXIETY
_____	_____	_____
_____	_____	_____
_____	_____	_____
_____	_____	_____

Irrational Fear

Fear and anxiety are often thought of as similar emotions. In fact, many psychologists use these terms interchangeably. However, people who experience high levels of both anxiety and fear report that there is a real difference between these two emotions.

While anxiety is related to the future, fear is an emotion that is grounded in the present. It is a reaction to something that is happening *right now*. For instance, if you were reasonably sure that a madman with a shotgun were to break into your house within the hour and threaten to kill you, you would probably feel unhealthily anxious. However, if he were with you right now and threatening you, that would be fear.

Irrational or unreasonable fear is destructive, bravery or courage is the pleasant alternative, and rational fear is the constructive alternative. It is reasonable to be afraid of someone who is threatening to kill you, but it is not reasonable to be afraid of standing in front of a group of people and giving a speech. The first situation is dangerous, the second is not.

You cannot feel the difference between rational and irrational fear—they both *feel* the same. The only way you can tell whether you are experiencing rational or irrational fear is by the use of your reason, your intelligence.

When you feel rational fear, you act to protect yourself and ensure your physical survival. Irrational feelings of fear will often lead you to behave defensively by putting up an emotional wall between yourself and others. Often you wall out those very people you need most for support and encouragement.

Irrational fear is frequently coupled with one of the other destructive emotions, as it is in this example: "This depression really scares the daylights out of me. I mean, I feel like something terrible is happening to me. My mind feels like mashed potatoes, and I get these unnerving feelings of being isolated and apart from people. These depressed feelings and sensations have me petrified. They could overwhelm me—they're dangerous.

This man is really experiencing two destructive emotions at the same time: depression and irrational fear. This is a common occurrence that makes it even more difficult to understand what you are feeling.

COURAGE	IRRATIONAL FEAR	RATIONAL FEAR
_____	_____	_____
_____	_____	_____
_____	_____	_____
_____	_____	_____

Destructive emotions are a waste of your time—and your life. Most people don't realize it, but they do not have to experience guilt, unwarranted fear, helplessness, or even depression. You have the power to release these emotional rascals and banish them from your life. It takes hard work, changes in your thoughts and behavior patterns, and most of all COMMITMENT, to say goodbye to destructive emotions.

The problem is that no one has taught you *how* to change these emotions to your advantage. You have gone to school to learn all sorts of things—but it is unlikely that anybody has taught you how to deal with your feelings in a tangible and positive way.

Other painful emotions, the constructive ones, need to be met head on and accepted as part of life. It's a natural part of the human condition to react to life with sadness, a sense of weakness, regret, healthy anxiety, rational fear, and yes, even anger. These feelings are your safety valve. Unlike destructive responses, they will quickly run their course and leave you a stronger person over the long haul.

Reacting in a healthy and constructive way to difficult circumstances does not mean that you never get upset or hurt. After all, you are not an unfeeling, detached, emotional robot. You were created a feeling person. But you were also designed as a thinking human being, a person with a brain—and most importantly, a person with the power of choice. You can learn to choose constructive responses to life and all that it brings. This process can begin NOW. Recovery doesn't have to wait for months and years. By working very hard at the new skills you will be learning, you can limit—and even eliminate—the occurrence of some destructive emotional responses.

To help you remember the destructive emotions and how they fit with your environment and your behavior, study the following chart. I recommend you copy it and place it in the back of your Voice Fighting Kit.

Understanding Your Emotions		
Source	**Constructive Emotions** *Destructive Emotions*	Behavior
Loss	**Sadness**	**Crying**
	Depression	*Lifelessness*
Mistake	**Remorse**	**Forgiveness**
	Guilt	*Self-Punishment*
Conflict	**Weakness**	**Self-Improvement**
	Helplessness	*Escape*
Violation	**Anger**	**Confrontation**
	Resentment	*Retaliation*
Threat	**Healthy Anxiety**	**Encounter**
	Unhealthy Anxiety	*Avoidance*
Feelings (danger)	**Rational Fear**	**Self-Protection**
	Irrational Fear	*Insulation*

Sorting Out Your Feelings

In order to learn how to minimize the influence of destructive emotions in your life, you must be able to recognize their existence. In order to do this you will need to keep an accurate record of your destructive emotions throughout the day. This will be done by adding a fourth column to your Voice Diary. These columns will be entitled: time, situation, destructive emotion, and Voice.

It is critically important that you devote time each day filling out this diary in order to understand your destructive emotions better. Once you know the difference between destructive emotions and their constructive counterparts, you can begin to become more precise in mentally grasping what happens to you when you feel "down," "bummed out," or are having a "rotten day."

It is also important to be able to label these emotions when they are happening, not a week later. To help you get on top of these emotions, it is extremely important to keep your Emotions Diary current. An example of how this diary looks is given below. You will want to keep your diary in your notebook and work on it every day.

Emotions Diary

Time	Situation	Destructive Emotion	Voice
9:00 A.M.	Slept in late	Resentfulness	Your stupid husband forgot to wake you up.
Noon	Friend coming for lunch	Helplessness	You can't stand being trapped in your own house—as long as she is here you won't be able to eat what you want.
3:00 P.M.	Pick up kids from school	Guilt	You should not have been late getting your kids from school
3:30 P.M.	Watching soaps	Depressed	You are really a bad mother—a totally worthless human being.
8:00 P.M.	Reading paper	Anxious	What if you are late again and someone kidnaps your children? You wouldn't be able to handle a tragedy like that.

| 8:15 P.M. | Reading paper | Fear | Do you feel all that anxiety right now? It is really dangerous and could hurt you. |

The first column in the example is used to record the time of the destructive emotion; the second records the situation; the third is the actual destructive feeling; and the fourth is the Voice. There may be times when you will not be able to confidently label your destructive emotion. In this case, you might want to amplify your situational description and leave the third column blank. Coming back to it later or having your support person help you can often show you which emotion you are dealing with. Continued practice will help you begin identifying the emotion immediately. Then you can rapidly identify the specific destructive feeling on the spot, you will be more confident about sorting out your feelings.

Of course there will be times when it is impossible to write down the emotion as you are experiencing it. You certainly can't write in your diary when you are driving your car, chatting with friends, or maybe even when you are feeling really depressed. In these cases, you need to write in your diary as soon as possible so that the details are fresh in your mind. Your small notebook will help here.

If you have been diligently practicing your stress reduction, it is now time to streamline it by shortening the amount of time it takes to release muscle tension. This can be done by concentrating on seven muscle groups instead of fifteen. Use the following suggestions to shorten your progressive relaxation.

1. *Right arm.* Hold your right arm out in front of you and bend your elbow just slightly. Now make a fist.

2. *Left arm.* Do the same.

3. *Face and scalp.* Do several different things all at the same time: wrinkle up your forehead, squint your eyes, wrinkle up your nose, bite down, and pull the corners of your mouth back.

4. *Neck and throat.* Bend your head forward and pull your chin downward toward your chest. You will feel a little bit of shaking or trembling in these muscles as you tense them.

5. *Upper torso.* Again, do several different things all at the same time: take a really deep breath and hold it, pull your shoulder blades back and together, and make your stomach as hard as you can.

6. *Right leg.* Lift your right leg up, straighten out your knee, and pull your toes up toward your face.

7. *Left leg.* Do the same.

Skills Checklist

☐ Continue relaxation/Natural Breathing

☐ Continue morning rituals (2)

☐ Continue evening rituals (2)

☐ Reread previous chapters

☐ Memorize the constructive-destructive emotions

☐ Keep a daily record in your Emotions Diary

6

Voice Analysis

A hundred cart-loads of worry wont pay an ounce of debt.

–ITALIAN PROVERB

At this point, you should be well aware that your problems do not stem from your situation, from people or circumstances, but from the way you *perceive* those people and events. It's your thinking—and not the outside world—that needs to be corrected.

So the key to recovery lies in changing your thinking patterns. As you know, that involves a lot of hard work and energy. That's because the Voice—the destructive self-talk that triggers your destructive emotions—just loves to get you so focused on your emotions and your body and so upset by your environment and the swirl of panic-related symptoms that you can't think straight enough to fight it.

How often has the Voice said this to you: "Look at you! You're panicked and upset, your body is a wreck, and your mind feels like mashed potatoes. You'll never get better."

That's a lie, and it's important you recognize that fact. The Voice is not that smart. It relies on strong-arm tactics, not logic. Its emotion-triggering lies revolve around a few key emotions and mindsets. In fact, the six destructive emotions discussed in chapter five are the traps that keep you from making progress in your life. And each of these six destructive emotions is brought about by a specific Voice message. Each message can be identified by a specific *key word*. Once you have learned the key words, you will be ready to use the Voice Fighting skills from chapter seven to nail the Voice on the spot.

Voice Messages and Key Words

If you don't feel entirely confident in identifying the six destructive emotions, then you need to review chapter five right now. As that chapter shows, the six destructive emotions are depression, helplessness, guilt, resentment, unhealthy anxiety, and irrational fear. These are the most common and the most destructive means the Voice uses to get your attention and thereby maintain your status as a victim.

You are going to learn how to use the Voice's tactics and turn them to your advantage. The six key words will let you tune in to the Voice and thereby find its secrets.

For example, let's say that you are bulimic, and you've just cleared out the refrigerator on a binge. Afterwards, you feel rotten, awful, and most of all *guilty*. The Voice is machine-gunning you with lies like "You did it now! You binged! That's terrible. You should not have done that!"

A bulimic untrained in Voice Analysis and Voice Fighting might be so bombarded with feelings and emotions that she couldn't even hear, much less fight, the Voice's lies. But using the information from this chapter, she can catch the Voice's key word within seconds. She can say to herself, "Since I'm feeling guilty, the Voice must be talking right now." After writing down what the Voice is saying to her, she will easily spot the *should* key word. She would instantly know that the Voice is trying to convince her that she is obligated to play by the rules and that any infraction is a major failure for her.

The Relationship Between Key Words and Emotions

Each key word is associated directly with a specific destructive emotion. These pairs always go together, so that knowing one will always point the way to the other one. The chart below shows how these are related.

The Key Word	The Destructive Emotion
Stand	Helplessness
Should	Guilt
Worthless [Me]	Depression
Worthless [Them]	Resentment
Tragedy	Unhealthy Anxiety
Danger	Irrational Fear

In order to make sense of these relationships, I want to spell out for you how each key word can lead to each destructive emotion. In the sections below, for each key word you will learn three things: the related emotion, the Voice's message associated with the key word, and the truth which opposes the lie of the key word.

Key Word: Stand (Tolerate, Cope, Handle)

The Emotion: Helplessness

The Voice's Message: "This thing that is happening to you right now is uncontrollable, awful, unstoppable. You can't stand it! You are trapped, hopeless, out of control forever."

The Voice wears you down, trying to convince you that you can't stand it anymore, you can't take it, something is driving you up the wall. The Voice tries to get you to believe that you are going to go crazy if you stay in this situation any longer.

With the Voice telling you that you can't stand it, you eventually begin to believe there really are certain things you "can't stand." This message becomes a self-fulling prophecy. When the Voice has convinced you that you can't stand something, you then leave the situation—and the Voice says to you, "See, I told you, you couldn't stand it."

When the Voice uses this key word with you, it will often try to confuse the difference between "leaving" and running away." You leave a situation because it is your choice to do so—you have decided that leaving is the better part of valor. Leaving the situation can be quite constructive and helpful.

Running away, however, is never helpful, because it is always done at the insistence of the Voice. There are many ways the Voice can get you to "run away" from something. The most obvious is to remove yourself physically from an uncomfortable situation. Less obvious, but just as common, is to run away emotionally. When you feel stress and fail to eat, this is a way to run away from the stress—and it generally works. Most people with anorexia "feel better" when they eat less. Binging is another way to run away. The bulimic often runs away twice: once from the stress of the situation (binging) and once from the guilt of the binge (purging).

It is very common for the Voice to use this key word with you when you feel physically uncomfortable. You have probably heard the Voice tell you that you "can't stand" any feelings of discomfort in your body. Many Deadly Dieters tell me they are keenly aware of body sensations that most other people give no thought to. For instance, you may be extremely sensitive to heat, light, and noise outside of your body, and also be extremely sensitive to internal sensations such as heartbeat, body temperature, fatigue, stomach irregularities, and dizziness.

A Canadian psychologist, G.D. Pulvermacher, has coined the term "discomfort dodging" to describe this low level of tolerance for discomfort. He defines "discomfort" as the psychological and physiological experience of disequilibrium—a definition that fits the sensations listed above. When you feel any of these sensations, the Voice will immediately jump in and say, "You can't stand these feelings," "You cannot control yourself," "You're trapped by this feeling and can't do anything about it."

When the Voice throws "stand" at you, it wants you to take the role of a victim. Feeling helpless and trapped leaves you with no options and no ability to make decisions. Consequently, you are at the mercy of other people, which makes you feel even more trapped and helpless. This game is just one continuous downward spiral.

Below are some examples of things the Voice may say to you when it is using this key word. Check those that sound familiar and add any that aren't listed.

- ☐ You can't stand being a fat person.

- ☐ You can't stand people asking how much you weigh.

- ☐ You can't stand the feeling of a full stomach.

- ☐ You can't stand being out of control.

- ☐ You can't stand looking in the mirror.

- ☐ You can't stand other people getting angry with you.

- ☐ You can't stand greasy foods.

- ☐ _____

- ☐ _____

- ☐ _____

The Truth: The truth is quite simple. In fact, it is so obvious that most people tend to miss it. It goes something like this: While the voice is telling you that you cannot stand something, *you are in fact standing it*. And you can really stand anything. You may not like it but you can stand it.

Anybody who has worked with Deadly Dieters can see this key word being used all the time. Some people, no matter how much good information they receive or how much support they have, will decide that it is no use.

It is common to hear a Deadly Dieter say, "I just can't stand my life anymore. No matter what I do, nothing helps. I just know that I will never get over this eating problem no matter what I do." This individual will *never* conquer her problem no matter how much great therapy she gets.

But the moment she can recognize this key word and change her thinking, she can begin to experience positive change in her life. "The Voice is trying to make me feel helpless by telling me that I can't stand being bulimic. But I know that it is lying to me. The truth is that I may not like having this problem, but I can stand it. And the sooner I begin to stand it and work on it, the sooner I will get on with my life."

In clinical medicine, we have clearly seen that people who decide that they can stand something (even though they don't like it) are the ones who are more likely to get well.

Those who convince themselves that they can't stand the pain are generally the ones who worsen.

When the Voice uses this key word with you, it will try to confuse the difference between "standing" and "liking." You can literally stand anything because you have most likely been standing it for a long time. Standing it doesn't mean you have to like it.

In fact, you can actually hate it. You can dread being in a situation. You can even wish that you had made a different choice. The point is that you are in the situation. The reality of the situation is that you may have to stay in it a little longer—but you *can* stand and survive what you greatly dislike.

Key Word: Should (Must, Ought, Have to)

The Emotion: Guilt

The Message: "You shouldn't have done that." The Voice wants you to believe that you have to run your life according to somebody else's rules. It wants you to feel obligated to someone or something.

To clarify this key word, it is important to remember that "should" has two different meanings in our language. There is the "should" of probability and the "should" of obligation. The should of probability means that if you mix two colors together you *should* get another color. You don't have to. You're not obligated to, but the laws of probability say it is very likely to happen.

The other meaning for "should" is the should of obligation. You *should* be nice to your mother. You *should* brush your teeth every day. You *should* be slender. It's this type of obligation that the Voice tries to use in order to get you hooked into guilt. The sense of obligation is always at the foundation of all guilt.

Sometimes the Voice will try to trick you by getting you to obey rules which can lead to worthwhile goals. For example, it might tell you, "you should work harder on conquering your eating disorder." This is definitely a worthwhile goal. But the insertion of the "should" key word by the Voice undermines the validity of the goal: the Voice has made it a mandatory obligation (and thus a potential source of guilt) instead of a reasonable and controllable choice that you have made.

Check off those examples that the Voice has used on you when it has been using "should" words.

☐ You are blowing it! You shouldn't do that.

☐ You should be able to get rid of this problem. You could, you know, if you really tried.

☐ You should have been more thoughtful of your sister at dinner tonight.

☐ _____

☐ You shouldn't have binged.

☐ _____

☐ You shouldn't have been so rude

☐ _____

☐ You should gain more weight so that your mother doesn't have to worry anymore.

☐ _____

The Truth: Since you are an adult you don't need to live by the rules. You need to learn how to make your own decisions in life. This may seem to run directly counter to all of your moral and ethical upbringing. And yet when you look at this truth more closely, you will see that it actually enhances your own moral values.

To understand this key word, you need to go back to that time when you were a very small child. When you were small, your parents gave you a lot of "should" messages. And there were very good reasons for doing this.

For example, you were probably told to stay away from fire, high places, deep water, and sharp knives. These "should" messages became rules that your parents hoped would keep you alive. These rules had physical survival value. If you found yourself near a hot stove, you could avoid pain, injury, or even death by following the rules. The pain that came from breaking the rules was a reminder that the rule had value and purpose.

As you became older, the rules became more socially oriented and endowed with social survival value. They still followed the same general format: "You should say 'please' and 'thank you'." "You should let your friends go first." "You should wash your hands before dinner." "You should share your toys with your friends."

Now that you have become an adult, you have collected thousands and thousands of "should" rules. These rules govern your life and show you which decisions to make, even though these "should" rules are not always an effective way of running your life. Yet, out of sheer habit, you continue to maintain these rules, keep them in your life, and use them to make decisions. I contend that no adult needs to follow "should" rules. Every adult can choose to throw these rules out and learn a better way to make decisions. That better way is called consequence of decision making.

Consequence decision making works like this. Whatever situation you are in, you ask yourself what the choices are. Then you estimate what the outcome of those choices are. The final step is to then decide which consequence you are willing to accept *without blame or excuse*.

Let's illustrate this with a simple example. Take the elementary rule, "You should be nice to your friends." Although most people would agree that this is a good rule, let's back off from it for a moment and examine the consequences for choosing to follow it—or not.

You have two choices: (1) you can be nice to your friends, or (2) you can choose not to be nice to your friends. Now, the probable result from being nice to your friends is that you will maintain or keep the friendships. The probable or expected result of not being nice to your friends is that you will lose those friends.

Your decision as an adult is based upon which consequence you are willing to accept *without blame or excuse*. If you're going to throw away the "should" rules for making decisions, then you will learn to make reasonable decisions based on consequences. For example, maybe after thinking about the two possible consequences above you decide to keep your friends. Then you will need to behave in such a way as to bring about this desired result.

At this point you have probably noticed something interesting—behavior motivated by consequences can be identical to behavior motivated by rules. You might behave in exactly the same way toward your friends whether you are following the "should" rule or whether you had made a choice based on consequences. So then what difference is there between the two styles of decision making? The difference becomes obvious when you make mistakes. If you have *chosen* to be nice to your friends and you do something thoughtless or insensitive, you will feel remorse—not guilt!

If you are nice to your friends because you *should* be nice, then your mistakes will make you feel guilty. Making decisions based on "should" will set you up for a lot of guilt. But when you choose to make decisions based on consequences, you can boot guilt out of your life.

The problem with choosing consequence decision making as a way of life is that "should" rules are very comfortable. If you are a person who lives a legalistic life based on rules, "should," and the expectations of others, then your life is highly predictable. And it is this drive for safety and security that the Voice uses to keep you locked into a life of "should," rules, and guilt. Guilt is the cost for safety, security, and predictability. And this is a high cost to pay for such comforts.

The better alternative, a life based on consequences, is a life of freedom and spontaneity, growth and surprises. But there is a cost for this choice: vulnerability, unpredictability, and risk taking. It is a way of life that buffets and tosses you about by many unforeseen events. In other words, you pay a cost whether you live a sheltered life of rules and regulations or a life of growth and freedom.

Nature teaches us the value of moving from the child mode of living to the adult mode of living. The larvae in its cocoon is safe, secure, and protected from its environment. However, if it stays in it too long, it will wither and die. It is meant to leave its place of security and fly away as a butterfly. This new life is one of freedom, but not without its dangers—any moment the butterfly can be eaten by a bird!

So when the Voice is laying a bunch of "shoulds" on you, it is important to remember that you're not obligated to do *anything* the Voice tells you to do. You may do anything if you choose to accept the consequences willingly—even when things go wrong. The Voice can also get quite tricky at this point. Sometimes it tells you to do something that seems reasonable. It might tell you, for example, to spend more time learning the techniques in this book. But remember: you NEVER do anything the Voice tells you. You must make your own decision whether you will work in this book or not, a decision based exclusively on your prediction of the consequences to do so.

One word of caution: the word "should" is not a key word when referring to another person. If the Voice tells you that someone else *should* be doing something, no key word is being used. Guilt is a destructive emotion which only applies to you.

Key Word: Worthless [Me] (Rotten, Terrible, No Good)

The Emotion: Depression

The Voice's Message: To get you depressed, the Voice will try to convince you that you are utterly worthless, through and through. But even this is not the entire message. The Voice doesn't just say what a terrible person you are; it tries to "prove" your worthlessness by connecting with a specific action or inaction. The Voice will tell you that your worth as a human being depends on your behavior.

Since nobody is perfect, your worth goes up and down like a YoYo according to this equation. When you do well, the Voice lets you feel worthwhile and good about yourself. But when you blow it, the Voice insists that your worth is nonexistent. By accepting the concept that your worth equals your behavior, you are forced to be a perfectionist in order to avoid depression. "If only I wouldn't screw up, then I wouldn't have to get depressed." And, of course, since you can't be perfect, you will continue to get depressed as long as you allow the Voice to use this key word with you.

This concept can easily be described as an equation: worth = behavior. It is a very difficult game to deal with because the Voice strongly reflects the values of our society. The worth = behavior idea is woven into the very fabric of American life. It is not difficult to see that society continually evaluates people's behavior based on a variety of standards. Some of the more common norms for judging worth are: wealth, education, power, fame, and beauty.

When we judge a person's worth by how much money he or she has, we are implying that the millionaire is "worth more" than the pauper. When we evaluate worth based on education, we are saying that the college professor is "worth more" than a high school dropout. When we accept power as a basis for worth, we can come to some fairly bizarre conclusions. Is a Mafia don really "worth more" than a petty criminal? We also evaluate people on their fame or status. Many people act as if an international rock star is "worth more" than a local musician struggling to make a living. But the most conspicuous form of evaluation is based on outward appearance. This is why the "beautiful" person seems to get all the breaks.

If an individual has a mixture of some of these qualities, he or she is usually accepted into the mainstream of society and can generally find friends and live a normal life. If that person has a large quantity of any of these five characteristics, he or she will probably be put on a pedestal and worshipped by others. Unfortunately, if a person has none of these qualities, he or she will more than likely end up in an institution somewhere.

A closer look at these criteria reveals that the last one, beauty, is a double standard. If a woman is not "pretty," it can be difficult for her to be given credit for any of the other four qualities.

If you're a woman working in an organization in which your advancement is based on other people's evaluations, you will do much better if you are very pretty. When is the last time you saw a woman executive in a major corporation who was not good looking? Women who are not pretty often find it easier to be successful in professions where their competence is not judged by other people's evaluations of what they look like. The sad part of this is that a man can be fat, bald, ugly, and obnoxious, but if he has enough money, people will love and accept him.

To fight the Voice with this key word is to swim upstream. It is to go against the present current of society. Even if you decide that being thin is not the most important thing in the world, others will bombard you with the notion that you must look or act a certain way.

See of any of these examples of *worthlessness* sound familiar to you.

☐ Only worthless people have eating disorders.

☐ You better not tell anyone about your problem or they will see how awful you really are.

☐ You're so rotten it's not even worth your effort to try changing yourself.

☐ The world would be better off without scum like you.

☐ If you weren't such an awful human being, you might be happier.

☐ You know that everyone around you is better than you.

☐ _____

☐ _____

The Truth: Your worth does NOT depend on what you achieve, and it certainly does not depend on your behavior. Rather than accepting the equation "worth = behavior" as a description of reality, you need to know that your worth is NOT equal to your behavior. Because you are alive, you have infinite worth! No matter how badly you mess things up, you are infinitely worthwhile. You were born with infinite worth and you cannot change that fact. You can't buy any more, you can't sell it, you can't give it away, and you can't barter it. You are stuck with the fact that you are infinitely worthwhile 24 hours a day, seven days a week. Regardless of what you do, you have infinite worth!

This is an extremely difficult concept for many people to understand. There are two sources which offer you help in digesting the notion that you have infinite worth. You can learn to accept your infinite worth from a philosophical, theological, or economics point of view. Whichever method helps to convince you of your worth, use it.

If you have a religious orientation, you can easily find evidence for your infinite worth. The Bible, for example, insists that you are made in the image of God. This is a supreme statement of your infinite worthfulness.

The philosophy of democracy also implies the theory of infinite worth. Since democracy demands that "all people are created equal" it must mean that equality is not measurable. If worth was measurable, then one person might have 100 units of worth. This would immediately suggest that somewhere someone else must have more or less than 100 units. If we all have the same amount of worth, then the only amount we can have is infinite—that theoretical place in mathematics where there are no numbers.

The next time the Voice tells you that you are a lousy, rotten, stupid human being because of something you have done, you need to remember the flaw in this key word. You can certainly say, "I really regret having done this stupid thing and hurting another human being, but I still have infinite worth." If you want to rid yourself of depression, leaving only sadness, then it is important that you understand this flaw right now.

Key Word: Worthless [Them] (Useless, Rotten, Unimportant)

The Emotion: Resentment, hatred, bitterness, hostility

The Voice's Message: When the Voice convinces you that another person is awful, terrible, or a no-good louse, then you are being set up for resentment. The Voice wants you to believe that the other person's behavior makes him a bad, worthless individual. Resentment is the flip side of depression. If you apply the worth = behavior concept to another human being, rather than to yourself, you will find yourself wanting to retaliate against that person. One of the clues that you are feeling resentment instead of anger is the use of name-calling and derogatory labels.

This key word is probably the least used by the Voice of Deadly Dieters. In fact, you may find it strange we have included this key word because you believe that you don't hate anyone. You may also be the type of person who never gets angry at people, no matter what they do. Even if this is the case with you, it is still wise for you to be aware of the potential of this key word. One of the more common experiences of people who come to my clinic is the emergence of resentment near the end of treatment. When other, more powerful key words begin to subside, it is not all uncommon for the Worthless [Them] to rear its head. If you are not expecting it, you may totally miss it and be baffled by what the Voice is saying to you. Or else you may be so shocked at its appearance that you let the Voice blast you with "shoulds," and you begin to feel guilty.

Many people have been confused about the relationship between depression and resentment. You have probably heard it said, "depression is anger turned inward." This is not true, since anger is constructive and resentment is destructive. It would be more accurate to say that depression is the worth = behavior equation turned inward, and resentment is the same equation turned outward.

Do any of the following examples of this key word look familiar to you?

☐ People who don't under-
stand you are awful.

☐ If he wasn't such an
idiot, he would be more
sympathetic to your eating
disorder.

☐ You're different from the
rest of these jerks you see
every day.

☐ _____

☐ You don't need garbage like
that in your life.

☐ _____

☐ Anyone who gives you a
hard time ought to be shot.

☐ _____

The Truth: Of course, the truth is identical to that of the previous key word. Regardless of what someone else does to you, he or she still has infinite worth. This doesn't mean that you have to ignore what has been done to you. Nor does it mean that you can't get angry at what has happened to you. You have the right to get mad when someone has violated your basic rights. You don't, however, have the right to retaliate in kind.

Another distinction can be seen, now, between resentment and anger. Resentment means you are judging and evaluating another person's worth based on what he or she has done to you. Anger indicates that you are confronting that other person's behavior. Resentment concentrates the worth side of the equation; anger concentrates on the behavior side.

This key word can be very abusive both toward yourself and toward others. But then this is a natural consequence of believing that worth = behavior. Remember the distortion of this key word when the Voice wants you to evaluate your own or someone else's performance. A person's worth is NOT equal to behavior. No matter what a person does, infinite worth is never diminished.

Of all the key words, this is the one which is most difficult for many of my clients to believe. The emotions we feel when we have been wronged are powerful and difficult to ignore. Many people have experienced feeling much better when they have been able to get back at someone who has hurt them. Remember, though, that feelings are extremely poor reasons for doing anything.

Key Word: Tragedy (Catastrophe, Calamity, Disaster)

The Emotion: Unhealthy anxiety

The Voice's Message: The format of this key word is generally, "What if such and such happens, then that would be a tragedy!" A typical example would be, "What if you lost control of your eating and blew up

like a blimp and everybody hated you—that would be a catastrophe."
Notice that these sentences have two parts: a "what if" and a "tragedy,"
The second part, the tragedy, is actually the most dangerous portion of
this message. It is the trigger that generates the unhealthy anxiety.

This message is like an iceberg, part of which is highly visible, part
of which is invisible. Since most of the iceberg mass is below the water-
line, it is this part which is dangerous to ships coming near it. Likewise
with the key word "tragedy." The "what ifs" don't really cause a problem.
It is the addition of the tragedy that makes them so destructive.

Generally speaking, tragedies for people with eating disorders tend
to center around embarrassment themes (other phobias also add the
"tragedy" of death). The embarrassment is most readily seen when the
Voice asks you what other people will think about what you decide to
do. You may spend much of your waking hours worrying about what
other people think. Of course, in reality very few people even bother to
think about what you do, but the Voice has convinced you that you are
constantly on stage and wherever you go and whatever you do people
are always watching you.

Maybe some of the following examples of this message are prominent in your life.

- [ ] What if you gained weight and looked ugly? What a tragedy that would be.

- [ ] If people found out you were not perfect, nobody would love you.

- [ ] What if someone found out about your eating disorder? You would be humiliated beyond description.

- [ ] What if you got locked up in the loony bin because someone realized how sick you really are.

- [ ] What a catastrophe it would be if you failed that exam.

- [ ] _____

The Truth: Since this key word has two lies, there are also two
truths. You must be able to tell the difference between them so that you
know what the Voice is telling you and how to respond. Since the "what
if" part is usually more visible than the tragedy part, this is where you
will want to begin. When you hear the "what if," you need to remember
that this is a distorted prediction, soon to be followed by the tragedy—
which is also distorted.

Let's look at the first flaw in the "what ifs." When the Voice is
"what-iffing" you, it is really doing more than making the suggestion that
something bad may happen. The Voice is actually saying, "I have it on
good authority that this awful thing will definitely happen to you. I know
there's a 99 percent chance that something bad will happen to you." Do

you see what the Voice is doing? It is giving you a guarantee that it can read your future. It is telling you it knows what will happen in your life.

Now you can see the error or the flaw in this claim. Nobody, including the Voice, can accurately predict the future. To get a true estimate of how well the Voice can do this, think about all the "what ifs" you've ever heard in your entire life. It has to be an incredibly big number. For the average person on the Deadly Diet this number could easily be in the tens of thousands. Now think of the number of times these "what ifs" have actually come true. You can probably count all of these events on one hand. Simple math will tell you that if there are thousands of *possible* occurrences and only a few *actual* occurrences, then the probability of something happening is extremely low.

The flaw in this first part of the game is: "The liklihood that an awful thing will happen to me is extremely low." In fact, the odds are in your favor that something awful will NOT happen. The odds are always working for you. It is important to respond to this flaw by reducing the mountain back down to its original molehill. You need to firmly believe the Voice cannot read the future!

Resisting this flaw has only limited effectiveness. No matter how far you reduce the probability, you will never get it to zero—one over something is never zero. If you have convinced yourself that a particular "what if" has a one in a million chance of occurring, the Voice will counter this response with, "Yeah, but this could be that one time." Embedded in this statement is a further notion: "And if this is that one time, it will be a tragedy."

It's at this point that you move to the second part of this message and deal with the flaw of definition. To do this you need to understand what the word "tragedy" really means. The concept of a tragedy was first fully developed by writers of ancient Greece. For the Greeks, a tragedy consisted of two elements: loss of control and personal awareness of this loss. In many of the Greek stories, people were put in situations in which they no longer had any control over their destiny. The individual was sometimes doomed to engage in certain repetitive behaviors forever. But that wasn't the tragedy. The tragedy existed because that individual was totally, consciously aware of his or her loss of ability to make choices.

You may remember the story of Sisyphus. In Greek mythology, he was a king of Corinth who was condemned forever to rolling a stone up a hill in Hades, only to have it roll down again on nearing the top. Many people think the tragedy in this story is the inability of Sisyphus to contol his own destiny. But the real tragedy was his human awareness of this loss of personal control. Every moment, every second of his drudgery, Sisyphus *knew* that he had no other choices. He knew that he had been stripped of his ability to make his own decisions. This story represents the ultimate in human tragedy. The genius of the Greeks realized there is nothing more tragic than knowing that you cannot make personal choices.

If we bring this idea of personal tragedy back to the real world you and I live in, we can quickly recognize that there is no such thing as a personal tragedy. No matter what happens, you can still think, act, and make choices. There are a few events that can keep you from doing that— a coma or death—but even these two things would not be personally tragic, because *you wouldn't be aware of them.*

Around the turn of the century there arose a way of looking at life called existentialism. Writers, novelists, and philosophers were saying that the essence of being human is *to act*. Making choices and acting on them ensures us of our humanity. The existentialists realized that choice and action were the exact opposite of Greek tragedy. They knew that as long as you were capable of choices and action you could not experience a tragedy in your life.

Of course, we can still admit sociological tragedies into human experience. An earthquake that kills 5000 people in Peru is a *sociological* tragedy. It is not a personal tragedy, because the people who died are not aware of the loss of life and the people who survived can still make choices and go on with life.

Once you recognize that there can be no personal tragedy for you, the supports are knocked out from under this key word. No matter how low the chances of something bad happening, you still have the ability to choose what to do about it. It would not be tragic, because no matter how bad it was, you would still be capable of making decisions and DOING SOMETHING!

Fortunately, nobody, including the Voice, can accurately predict the future. Remember that this message always has two parts. The flaw in the first lies in the overblown probabilities of the "what if" statement— this "what if" statement is really making reference to a very low probability event. The last person in the world to blow up like a blimp is a person on the Deadly Diet. Nevertheless, no matter how low the chances of such an event happening, it still could! If it did, it would merely be unfortunate, inconvenient, or uncomfortable—not tragic. It would not be tragic, because no matter how bad it was, you would still be capable of making decisions and taking action to correct the situation.

Key Word: Dangerous (Unsafe, Treacherous, Frightening)

The Emotion: Irrational fear

The Voice's Message: The Voice first tries to get you to tune into any type of discomfort in your body—whether physical sensations or emotions. When you become aware of what is happening, the Voice then tells you that what's going on inside of you is dangerous. *"These feelings you're experiencing are scary and dangerous. They could really hurt you!"*

The Voice loves to use this key word immediately after using one of the other ones. For instance, when you are feeling depressed, the Voice will point to this feeling and try to tell you that you need to be afraid of it. So now, in addition to depression, you have a bonus emotion: irrational fear. The Voice enjoys getting you so absorbed in and terrified of destructive emotions that you become absolutely certain they can destroy you.

It is difficult to feel irrational fear by itself, because irrational fear is the fear of what's going on inside of you. When you are feeling irrational fear, there is a good possibility that another destructive emotion is also present.

Sally felt depressed one afternoon because she had just had a terrific binge that morning. It was her biggest binge in six months. The Voice had really gotten a foothold in her life and was telling her what a rotten person she was for doing such an awful thing. When she became aware that she was feeling intense depression, everything seemed to get worse. She now felt a terrible fear of something that she couldn't put her finger on. After much writing, she discovered that the Voice was telling her how dangerous her depression was. By accepting this lie, Sally was now feeling fear in addition to her depression.

This message acts like a parasite because it often lives off one of the other messages. But the Voice can also use this key word with other triggers. Any bodily sensation is eligible to become a trigger for irrational fear. One client of mine told me of a fear that had gripped her all week. No matter how hard she tried, she could not identify the object of her fear. When I asked her to try to remember the last time this had happened to her, she replied, "Oh, the same time last month." She had not even thought of considering her own bodily functions as a target for this key word.

Other common triggers are fatigue and sickness. For example, the Voice can get you to feel irrationally afraid when you are feeling tired. When you're very tired the Voice might say to you, "Uh oh, watch out, do you feel that? It's dangerous." Now in addition to feeling tired, you feel fearful.

Feeling sick or having a fever can also trigger off this key word. Since you already feel bad from the illness, it is often difficult to switch gears mentally and become aware of the presence of the Voice and the associated key word.

You may have noticed by now that this game points up a significant difference between rational and irrational fear. Rational fear is always directed away from you; irrational fear is directed inward. For years, the mental health community was not aware of this and was puzzled by people's irrational fear. When the subject was brought up, the well-meaning therapist would discuss all of the things in the person's life that could possibly be perceived as dangerous. The fear object was being looked for in the wrong place. Irrational fear always is concerned with what is happening inside, not outside of you.

Some sample messages of how this key word is used:

☐ You're feeling really light-headed right now, and you know how dangerous that can be.

☐ This feeling of extreme anxiety could really hurt you.

☐ These heart palpitations you are having now could kill you.

☐ You better watch out because this helplessness is awfully scary.

☐ It is really awful when you feel bloated.

☐ _____

The Truth: The truth is quite simple: there are no dangerous feelings. Feelings may be painful or hurtful, but they are not dangerous. Remember that irrational fear generally focuses itself on something inside of you. The Voice tries to convince you of something that is simply not true: namely, that those feelings and sensations inside of you can hurt you and destroy you. The fact is, they may hurt you, but they cannot destroy you.

The table on the next page summarizes the relationship between the situation, the key word (message), the destructive emotion, and the destructive behavior. The last column has the Truth, which you will be using in the next chapter to fight the Voice.

At this point I would not expect you to believe the Truths. If you did, you wouldn't need to be reading this book. All you need at this point is to understand the Truths. Belief will come later, after you have spent time Voice Fighting.

The words in column two which are emphasized are the *key words*. You will need to memorize these words because they will instantly identify for you the lies that the Voice is trying to force down your throat.

Homework

1. Your ability to defeat the Voice and fight back against its lies will depend on how well and how fast you can identify these six key words. To assist you in this, you want to put a copy of the Key Words Summary chart in your Voice Fighting Kit. You can either reduce the chart in the book or copy it in by hand. I recommend putting it at the back of the set of index cards.

2. With the six key words in your mental toolbox, you are now a Voice detective. Your feelings and emotions can point you toward the key

Key Word Summary

Source	Message	Emotion	Behavior	Truth
Conflict	You can't *stand* it.	Helplessness	Escape	**I have been standing it all my life.**
Mistake	You *should (not)* do that.	Guilt	Self-punishment	**I can make my own decisions be-cause I am a responsible adult.**
Loss	You are *worthless* because...	Depression	Lifelessness	**No matter what I do, I still have infinite worth.**
Violation	They are *worthless* because...	Resentment	Revenge	**No matter what they do, they still have infinite worth.**
Threat	Something bad will happen and that will be a *tragedy.*	Unhealthy Anxiety	Avoidance	**Nothing can happen to me which will keep me from making decisions.**
Feelings	These feel-ings you are having are *dangerous.*	Irrational Fear	Insulation	**Even though these feel-ings are un-comfortable, they can make me stronger.**

words. They can give you an emotional "hook," something you can grab onto as you try to sort through the barrage of feelings and get to the heart of the lies. As you get more efficient at spotting the key words, you will be better prepared to then begin Voice Fighting.

To help learn these six key words, the following exercise gives you real-life examples of how the key words might be used. For each of the twelve statements, fill in the appropriate key word.

1. _____Your revolting father doesn't have any right to hassle you about your weight.

2. _____It's *really* scary when you are feeling so self-destructive.

3. _____You're an awful person because you lied to your spouse about your eating habits.

4. _____You just *have* to get over this eating problem of yours.

5. _____What a calamity if you had this eating problem for the rest of your life.

6. _____Other people's comments about how you look just drive you up the wall.

7. _____You shouldn't have given in to your urge to binge and purge.

8. _____You just can't tolerate feeling bloated and fat.

9. _____It would be a catastrophe if you ever put on more weight.

10. _____Fat people are despicable.

11. _____This anxiety is unsafe and could make you crazy!

12. _____You're a rotten person because of the pain you cause your family.

Answers:

1. Worthless [Them]	5. Tragedy	9. Tragedy
2. Dangerous	6. Stand	10. Worthless [Them]
3. Worthless [Me]	7. Should	11. Danger
4. Should	8. Stand	12. Worthless [Me]

3. Continue your Voice Diary but switch to a two-column format. The left column is labelled "Voice" and the right column is labelled "me."

Continue to write what the Voice says in the left column. When you spot a key word, circle it and write the truth in the right-hand column.

4. Put the following chart that you can xerox and put on the first page of your wire-bound index cards (Voice Fighting Kit). The inside front cover will be used for something else.

Key Word Chart	
Generic Key Word	My Key Word(s)
Stand	
Should	
Worthless [Me]	
Worthless [Them]	
Tragedy	
Danger	

Put the key words which the Voice uses with you in the right-hand column. Some people never hear the Voice tell them they can't "stand" something, for instance. To them the Voice says they can't handle it or can't cope with it. Whatever word or words the Voice uses that mean the same as those words in the left column, you want to watch for. By having them in the right column, you will be more able to spot them.

5. Once again, you can streamline your progressive relaxation by working now on only four muscle groups. This is done by combining the tension-release of hands and arms; by combining legs and feet (try pressing down with both heels and lifting your toes up); by combining neck, throat, face, and scalp; and continuing with the usual procedure for your upper torso.

Skills Checklist

☐ Continue relaxation/Natural Breathing

☐ Continue morning rituals (2)

☐ Continue evening rituals (2)

☐ Reread previous chapters

☐ Memorize the constructive-destructive emotions

☐ Keep a daily record in your Emotions Diary

7

Voice Fighting

The voice is nothing but beaten air.

—SENECA, c. 62 A.D.

This chapter begins Phase III in your Voice Training by teaching you how to finally fight back against the Voice and its dominating influence in your life. Your goal is to learn the skill of Voice Fighting so well that you can practice it automatically and easily. Then, whenever destructive emotions begin to take over your life, you can regain control of your life by using the skill of Voice Fighting.

Unfortunately, as you learn to fight the Voice, it will become sneakier and nastier in its attempt to keep you as its slave. But with Voice Fighting, you can always stay one step ahead of the Voice. Remember that your eating disorder is not the real problem. The real problem is being out of control—and this happens because the Voice is running your life. Your ability to control your eating disorder depends on your effectiveness in fighting the Voice.

If you have been practicing your Voice Training skills with a partner or therapist, you will find that Voice Fighting is also a skill more easily learned with another person. It is often helpful to have another person play your part while you role-play the Voice. Since your Voice is not the other person's Voice, he or she will not feel as intimidated by what your Voice is saying as you would. This makes it easier for your partner to use the correct response. After a few practice attempts you can reverse roles, with your partner being your Voice and you practicing Voice Fighting. But when you practice Voice Fighting with someone else, it is important to agree to stop in midstream if you need to think of what to say or to correct an inappropriate response. Partner practice is the time to make mistakes and stop to correct them.

Voice Fighting Categories

When the Voice speaks to you (whether you are aware of it or not), you have only four possible responses available to you: Agreement, Distraction, Recitation, or Disagreement. Two of these responses are constructive ones; two are destructive. From another point of view, two of the responses deal with the "content" of the Voice message, while the other two are responses dealing with the "process" of what the Voice is doing to you. The following diagram illustrates how these four responses are related to each other.

	CONSTRUCTIVE	DESTRUCTIVE
PROCESS	RECITE	IGNORE
CONTENT	DISAGREE	AGREE

Agreement

The least effective response is to agree with everything the Voice says. This response has absolutely no redeeming value! It is a devastating response for you because it generates destructive emotions. Overwhelming you with these destructive emotions is exactly what the Voice wants. Agreement is the response you have been using most of your life, so it will be difficult at first to stop this habit.

This response is also the "default" response. If you are not actively engaged in using one of the other three responses, you are automatically using this response. There is no fifth response—you cannot *not* use one of these four responses with the Voice.

When the Voice tells you that you are fat and you agree with this observation, you are using this response. When you eat fewer calories because the Voice tells you to lose weight, you are using this response. When you procrastinate because the Voice says you will fail anyway, you are using this response.

To agree with the Voice at any time, no matter how reasonable it sounds, is always to be defeated and to feel helplessness, guilt, depression, resentment, unhealthy anxiety, or irrational fear.

Distraction

Although agreeing with the Voice is never effective, trying to ignore the Voice is only sometimes effective. Some of the time it works by taking your mind off the Voice. When you are concentrating on other things, you don't have to pay attention to the Voice. But this second response does not work for very long. It is only a short-term solution for dealing with the Voice. After the distraction time is over, the Voice comes back with a vengeance, making your life even more miserable than ever.

You will notice that distraction is called a "process response" on the chart above. In other words, it makes no difference what the Voice is saying to you, you merely tune it out. This response is concerned only with the fact that the Voice is talking to you, not with what it is saying.

This response sometimes functions as a combination of tuning out and running away. Most Deadly Dieters admit that they are often incredibly busy. The worst time for them is when nothing is happening. Boredom becomes a thing to be feared, because that is when the eating behavior (really the Voice) is the most uncontrollable.

At times when you are using Distraction, it can feel like being in the eye of a hurricane. Even though the eye is calm and peaceful, you know deep down that it won't last very long. Soon the storm will hit you with its full fury when the eye passes. So with the Voice. The longer this response is used by itself, the more powerful the Voice seems when it returns. Even when you are doing well several months from now, you will still be tempted to forget Voice Fighting and spend much of your time attempting to ignore it. The longer you do this, the bigger the setback you will eventually have. Since the Voice knows this, it will encourage you to "take time off and enjoy yourself." It knows that the longer you ignore it, the more setbacks you will have. This makes it possible for the Voice to regain all the power it has lost.

Because this response is so short-lived, it is essentially useless—by itself—for your long-range goal of defeating the Voice. When used in combination with Recitation and Disagreement, however, it can be a good tool against the Voice.

Many people bounce back and forth between these first two responses. After agreeing with the Voice, they ignore it by becoming real busy.

When the distraction response wears off, the person is right back to using the first response. You may find yourself in this cycle and wonder what else you can do to make yourself feel better. The next two responses will give you two more skills to be used in your fight against the Voice.

Recitation

Like the distraction response, this response deals with what the Voice is doing to you. Rather than reply to the specific message, you treat the Voice as you would any obnoxious person who is harassing and abusing you. When an offensive person is treating you badly, you tell him to "buzz off." You do the same thing with the Voice, except that your language is as strong as you can make it. If you find yourself getting angry at the Voice (an emotion often difficult for Deadly Dieters), you are probably using this response correctly.

Too often people tell the Voice to go away in such a defensive manner that it only reinforces their own sense of weakness. Remember, you are not having a tea party with the Voice or even engaging it in a debate. Rather, you are locked into a life-and-death struggle for your very existence.

To use this response efficiently, it is helpful to have a canned phrase in the back of your mind. This canned phrase needs to be as strong as you can make it. Right now, take a few moments off from reading this book and close your eyes. With your eyes closed, think of the most awful, vicious, nasty, mean, and rotten phrase you can think of to use as your recitation response. Since only you and the Voice will ever hear this phrase, don't be afraid to throw in a few words that you would never think of using in polite company. When you have found your phrase, open your eyes and continue reading.

The first time you use this response, it may shock you. The shock will back the Voice off momentarily. Some people find this original response so powerful that they want to use it all the time. But you must avoid this temptation, because this response has a built-in flaw: the more you use it, the weaker it becomes. You must use this response with discretion and caution. It works best when it is used in conjunction with the next response.

Disagreement

Disagreement is always the preferred response to any message from the Voice. The more you use it, the more powerful and strong you become and the weaker the Voice becomes. However, there are certain guidelines that must be followed in order to be successful in Voice Fighting.

The most important thing to remember is that you cannot successfully fight the Voice unless you know what it is saying. Some people report fighting and fighting with the Voice to no avail. Upon further examination, it inevitably becomes apparent that these individuals are not really hearing what the Voice is saying. Consequently, Voice Fighting for them is like fighting shadows. This is why the first two phases of Voice Training are so important. If you cannot hear the Voice or analyze its message into its component parts, then it will be literally impossible for you to fight back.

When the Voice hassles you, it can only do so in one of three ways. It can make a statement of fact, make a demand, or ask a question. You can deal with each of these three situations by learning the Basic Voice Fighting Response (BVFR) and several simple interrogation techniques.

The Basic Voice Fighting Response

The Voice will always try to control you by playing one of its games with you. To fight back means using the five-step Basic Voice Fighting Response: (1) identifying the destructive emotion, (2) naming the destructive behavior, (3) specifying the message, (4) stating the Truth, and (5) arguing with the Voice. If these steps sound familiar, it is because the first four are identical to the information you are currently recording in your Voice Diary. Since you already know the first four steps, the BVFR will be easy to learn.

If these five steps are carefully followed each time the Voice makes your life miserable, you will be able to quickly eradicate it from your life. Let's take a closer look at this five-step BVFR.

Step 1: Identify the Emotion

When you first begin to fight the Voice, you will usually become aware of its presence by the existence of a destructive emotion. Eventually, you will be able to identify the message even before the destructive emotion hits you. Either way, you have the information to begin fighting back.

If you are still a little shaky in identifying the emotions and the messages, you'll need to review chapter six on the key words and emotions. The key here is that the Voice actually plays into your hands by making you feel depressed or guilty. When you can correctly identify the destructive emotion, you then have the ammunition to fight back by responding to the Voice.

"Voice, you're trying to make me feel [*emotion*]"

Step 2: Name the Destructive Behavior

It is important to identify the behavior so that you can anticipate what the Voice wants you to do. Often the Voice wants you to be so wrapped up in emotion that you can't see where it is leading you. Remember that emotions are a process and never exist in isolation. They are preceded by thoughts and followed by behavior. As you begin to see what the Voice wants you to do, you can decide whether it is worth doing.

Correctly recognizing what the Voice wants you to do gives you a broader perspective than the emotional pain which you presently feel. You begin to see the connection between the pain and the destructive behavior. Rather than taking responsibility for binging or purging, you blame it on the Voice. This frees you up to focus on yourself and what is really in your own best interests.

After you have replied to the Voice by naming the emotion, your next reply will follow the formula: "You're trying to get me to [*behavior*]."

Step 3: Specify the Message

It is not enough to automatically put a label on what the Voice is saying to you. Identifying the key word is just the beginning of finding out what the Voice is really saying to you. After all, there are hundreds of ways for the Voice to tell you that you are worthless. Once you have put your finger on the exact message, you need to listen to the specifics. At this point, you will probably discover that the Voice is telling you about a specific event related to a real Voice Trigger in your environment.

With practice, as you begin to readily identify the Voice's precise message, you will also learn to anticipate when and where the Voice will strike next. To do this, your next reply needs to be: "You're telling me [*message*]. "

Step 4: State the Truth

Long ago someone said, "The truth shall set you free." This is exactly why you want to emphasize the Truth while the Voice is lying to you and getting you all riled up. I don't expect you to believe the truth when you first begin using it. If you did, you wouldn't need the techniques in this book. Your goal at this point is to merely understand the explanations in the previous chapter. The bridge between understanding and belief is called *repetition*.

When you have finished this step, you have just taken apart the lie which the Voice has tried to beat you with. After you have paraphrased the Voice's message, you say: "The truth is [*Truth*]."

Step 5: Argue, Argue, Argue

This last step is the one that gives power to your fighting. The three arguments you will use are all variations of the flaw. They embellish the flaw and hammer home the lies that the Voice has been feeding you. And this step hits the Voice three times for every one time it tries to hassle you. So, in this sense, the odds are nicely in your favor. But you must be adequately prepared before arguing with the Voice. To argue against the Voice before this step would be like lacing up a pair of heavy boots, closing your eyes, and stepping into the ring with Muhammad Ali—you'd get killed.

Some people, on the other hand, never even try to get in the ring because they are convinced they cannot win a battle with the Voice. (This, of course, is another sneaky Voice trick.) This idea is nonsense. After all, you are flesh and blood, and the Voice is imaginary and fictitious. You must win, if you follow the five-step Basic Voice Fighting Response.

To help you in finding your three good arguments, I will give you ten sample arguments for each key word later in this chapter. You may use these samples, alter them in any way, or use your own arguments. You must always use what works best for you!

To effectively use the BVFR, you will need to be very structured. This is accomplished by diligently following all five steps. If the Voice tells you how "fat" you are and that this makes you a terrible person, you can reply like this:

1. "Voice, you're trying to make me feel depressed."

2. "You're trying to get me to be lifeless."

3. "You're telling me that I'm an awful person because you think I'm fat."

4. "The truth is that no matter how I look I have infinite worth!"

5a. "Even if I were fat I would still have infinite worth."

5b. "I'm getting really tired of you trying to make me feel depressed all the time."

5c. "If I don't let you get me depressed, I'll just be that much stronger to fight back against you."

Application

The Voice is like the Wizard of Oz. You remember when Dorothy and her companions finally came before the awful, terrible wizard? A curtain was accidentally flung aside, revealing a tiny, frightened little man who used illusion to put fear into the hearts of those who were stronger than him. Well, that is exactly how the Voice works on you. Since it knows that you are stronger and must eventually destroy it, the illusion it creates that you are weaker is its most effective way of controlling you. By the very nature of illusion, you cannot, without special training, know you are being fooled. Have you ever watched a good magician destroy reality and convince you that things are different than they really are? These illusions are fun as long as you know they are tricks. It is quite different when you become convinced the trickery is real. Don't let the Voice convince you that its cheap parlor tricks are part of the real world. Your intelligence and rationality must always be the final word in measuring the strength of the Voice.

The Voice will pull every trick in the book to get you off the track. For instance, it will try to get you arguing perpetually, so that you feel like you are running in a circle. To avoid useless repetition, you will need to learn when to use your other two responses—Recitation and Distraction.

You will find that when you begin using your basic Voice Fighting response, the Voice will try to quickly switch to another key word, "worthless [me]," and just as you get to step 3 or 4 the Voice will start telling you that you should not have acted as you did toward your friend. This confusing tactic must be handled carefully and slowly. Rather than attend to this new key word immediately, finish fighting the one you are currently on. Then, when you have finished with the three arguments, begin fighting the new key word. "Now what were you saying to me, Voice? Oh, yeah. You were trying to make me feel guilty. You are trying to get me to punish myself. . . ."

Just when you are in the middle of fighting this new key word, the Voice will do one of two things. It will either try to throw in other key words, or it will go back to the previous key word and attempt to get you running in circles. At this point you have two choices, depending on what the Voice actually does:

1. If the Voice goes to a new key word, you just finish up the one you are on and then start fighting the new one.

2. If, however, the Voice tries to get you to go back to a key word that you have already dealt with, you need to change tactics. If you don't do this, you could find yourself on a merry-go-round, fighting the same key words, nonstop, for the rest of your life.

Whenever the Voice starts to repeat itself, you need to stop using the Disagreement response and begin to use the Recitation response. In other words, you disregard what the Voice is saying to you and use your canned phrase. For instance, the Voice might use the *worthless [me]* key word with you, followed by the *should* key word, followed by the *worthless [me]* again. When this happens, you need to immediately use your Recitation response: "Now wait a minute, Voice. I've already fought that key word with you. So why don't you just buzz off and leave me alone!" (or whatever phrase you have chosen).

Of course, when you use your canned response, it is highly unlikely that the Voice will say, "Okay, I'll leave you alone." It is more likely that it will increase its efforts to upset you. It may even get nastier. Regardless of what it says, you again repeat your canned phrase. If the Voice still hassles you, repeat it one more time. This repetition of a canned response is called the "broken record" technique in assertion training. Of course, you could conceivably continue this response forever. That is why you will limit yourself to only three recitation responses.

Unfortunately, the Voice will probably not give up just because you stop using your Recitation response. If it still hassles you after you have used your canned response three times, proceed to Distraction. Deliberately ignore the Voice and all of its stupid comments. By fighting it and telling it where to go, you have paid your dues and are entitled to not pay attention to the Voice. When you do this, try to find something pleasant and enjoyable to do. "Goodbye, Voice! I've said all I have to say. You can go jump in a swamp—I'm going to go for a walk." Of course, if the Voice starts up again at a later time, you need to start all over again with Disagreement.

Voice Fighting Kit

It is important that you do not try to memorized this Basic Voice Fighting Response. Even if you knew every word cold, your mind would still go blank at the worst possible moment and then the Voice would have you. Better that you have a way to cheat for remembering what to say to the Voice.

The next thing you will put into your Voice Fighting Kit will be the Voice Fighting Decision Tree on the following page. (To order a packet of materials sized to fit into a set of wire-bound index cards, write to me at the California Clinic, 3838 Watt Avenue, Suite C-303, Sacramento, CA 95821, or call 916-488-3772.) This flow chart shows you exactly what to do at any given time. You can either copy it onto the inside front cover or else have the page copied and reduced to fit the inside front cover.

You now have this chart on the inside front cover of your Voice Fighting Kit and your Personal Key Words Chart right below it on the first page. On the next page—actually the top and bottom pages immediately following the Voice Fighting Decision Tree—put the first of six guidelines for Voice Fighting.

Voice Fighting Decision Tree

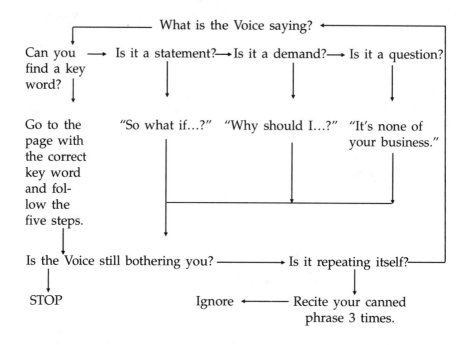

1. Distraction
2. Affirmation

Key Word: Stand, Handle, Tolerate, etc.

SOURCE: Conflict

1. Voice, you're trying to make me feel *helpless*.

2. You're trying to get me to *run away*.

3. You're telling me that I can't _____. . . .

4. The Truth is that I have been standing it all my life.

5. (Pick 3 arguments from the list below.)

　　If the Voice repeats the Key Word,
　　　A. Use your Canned Phrase, then
　　　B. Use Distraction

—————————Top page ↑ Bottom page ↓ —————————

Arguments

1. I may not like it, but I can deal with it.

2. What's happening to me now cannot make me feel trapped—only giving in to you, Voice, can do that.

3. I am strong and can control myself in any situation.

4. I have handled myself well in situations like this before.

5. The reason I am not trapped and helpless is because I can leave this situation any time I want to.

6. Agreeing with you, Voice, will only make me feel more powerless and miserable.

7. By allowing you to make me feel trapped, Voice, you deny me my freedom.

8. I refuse, Voice, to allow you to convince me of something so stupid and absurd—namely, that I am a helpless victim.

9. Other people don't feel helpless because they don't agree with you Voice.

10. If I run away from this situation now, things will only get worse and I will allow you, Voice, to have more power over my life.

When you have completed this page, continue until you have finished the pages for the rest of the key words.

Key Word: Should, Ought, Must, etc.

SOURCE: Mistake

1. Voice, you're trying to make me feel guilty.

2. You're trying to get me to punish myself.

3. You're telling me that I _____ (not). . . .

4. The Truth is that I can make my own decisions because I am a responsible adult.

5. (Pick 3 arguments from the list below.)

    If the Voice repeats the Key Word,
    A. Use your Canned Phrase, then
    B. Use Distraction

————————————Top page ↑ Bottom page ↓ ————————————

Arguments

1. I am going to substitute the words "will" or "choose" for the word "should."

2. I am an adult and can decide for myself what is right or wrong.

3. I now realize that I only feel guilty when you try to confuse fantasy and reality.

4. Guilt is one of your tricks to keep me dependent upon the unrealistic expectations of other people.

5. Even though I might wish that things were different, I can now recognize that I need to accept reality as it is.

6. I am not responsible for the feelings of other people.

7. I refuse to allow either you, Voice, or other people to guilt load me.

8. If I have really—objectively—hurt another person, I will apologize; otherwise I will not accept that monkey.

9. I can only overcome guilt by actively fighting you, Voice—even though you tell me I can't win.

10. If I don't want to feel guilty, I don't have to—all I need to do is fight back against you, Voice.

Key Word: Worthless, Rotten, No Good, etc.

[ME]

SOURCE: Loss

1. Voice, you're trying to make me feel *depressed*.

2. You're trying to get me to be *lifeless*.

3. You're telling me that I'm _____ because . . .

4. The Truth is that no matter what I do, I still have infinite worth.

5. (Pick 3 arguments from the list below.)

   If the Voice repeats the Key Word,
   - A. Use your Canned Phrase, then
   - B. Use Distraction

————————————Top page ↑ Bottom page ↓ ————————————

Arguments

1. No one or nothing can make me feel depressed—only agreeing with you, Voice, can do that.

2. Depression can be totally controlled by what I say to you, Voice.

3. No matter what I do, I am still a worthwhile person.

4. I allow myself to feel depressed by agreeing with you, Voice, when you tell me that I am a no-good person.

5. I am a wonderful, delightful, and lovable person merely because I am alive.

6. If other people put me down, I do not have to agree with their remarks.

7. Only you, Voice, can put me in the pit; only I can get myself out.

8. My depression will continue until I begin to vigorously fight you, Voice.

9. By keeping me depressed, you have total control over me—I refuse to allow this to happen!

10. It is okay for me to feel sad or discouraged without getting depressed.

Key Word: Worthless, Rotten, No Good, etc.
[THEM]

SOURCE: Violation

1. Voice, you're trying to make me feel *resentful*.

2. You're trying to get me to *retaliate*.

3. You're telling me that he or she is _____ because . . .

4. The Truth is that no matter what they did to me they still have infinite worth.

5. (Pick 3 arguments from the list below.)

   If the Voice repeats the Key Word,
   A. Use your Canned Phrase, then
   B. Use Distraction

——————————Top Page ↑ Bottom Page ↓ ——————————

Arguments

1. Other people are allowed to make mistakes.

2. No matter what a person does to me, they still have infinite worth.

3. Voice, you only want me to be resentful so that I will eventually cut off all human support and caring.

4. I can be angry without being resentful and full of hatred.

5. You lie when you tell me, Voice, that the way to get things done with other people is to retaliate so they won't hurt me again.

6. The more hatred you allow me to feel, the more self-destructive my own life becomes.

7. All of these resentful feelings are really making me weak and not strong as you would have me believe, Voice.

8. The only person I will allow myself to feel hatred toward is YOU!!

9. Voice, you are my worst enemy and the collection of all evil in the world.

10. Anger can be constructive and maturing if I learn how to handle it properly.

Key Word: Tragedy, Catastrophe, Awful, etc.

SOURCE: Threat

1. Voice, you're trying to make me feel *unhealthy anxiety*.

2. You're trying to get me to *avoid* things.

3. You're telling me that something bad is going to happen to me and that would be _____.

4. The Truth is that nothing can happen to me which will keep me from making choices.

5. (Pick 3 arguments from the list below.)

   If the Voice repeats the Key Word,
   - A. Use your Canned Phrase, then
   - B. Use Distraction

———————————Top page ↑ Bottom page ↓ ———————————

Arguments

1. It is reasonable to say "what if"; it is not reasonable to anticipate a personal tragedy or catastrophe.

2. Nothing bad will happen if I will just stop agreeing with you, Voice.

3. Even if something bad does happen, I can still act as a mature, responsible adult.

4. The worry is always worse than the actual event.

5. I can choose to stop worrying if I want to because worry is merely agreement with you, Voice.

6. I am and always will be in control; it is only you telling me that I am going to lose control.

7. I have always performed well and always will perform well in a crisis.

8. I can develop a plan to deal with anything!

9. Voice, you keep trying to trick me by insisting that a low probability event has a very good chance of happening.

10. If I allow myself to agree with you, I will only increase my chances of feeling misery and unhappiness.

Key Word: Dangerous, Scary, Frightening, etc.

SOURCE: Feelings

1. Voice, you're trying to make me feel *irrational fear*.

2. You're trying to get me to *insulate* myself.

3. You're telling me that these feelings are _____ and can destroy me.

4. The Truth is that even though these feelings are uncomfortable they can make me stronger.

5. (Pick 3 arguments from the list below.)

If the Voice repeats the Key Word,
   A. Use your Canned Phrase, then
   B. Use Distraction

——————Top Page ↑ Bottom Page ↓ ——————

Arguments

1. Feelings cannot destroy anyone—especially me.

2. If I want to get rid of this irrational fear, all I have to do is to fight you.

3. One of your lies is that if I don't insulate myself, other people will just use me as a doormat.

4. If this fear is rational, then it is normal and appropriate.

5. I refuse to let you, Voice, get me so irrationally afraid that I cannot think.

6. You're the source of all my irrational fears, Voice, so I've decided to fight you with all of my strength.

7. I am stronger than you, Voice. I'm going to win—you're going to lose.

8. I am not responsible for this irrational fear—it comes from agreeing with you.

9. Without you around I would never have to be unreasonably afraid anymore.

10. I am tired of being afraid of things that cannot hurt me.

Interrogating the Voice

Fighting the Voice is going to get easier for you the more you do it. If you continue to use your Voice Fighting Kit, you will find yourself winning most of the fights with the Voice. Now even though the Voice is cruel, it is not stupid. As you get stronger, it knows its days are numbered. Eventually it will realize that every time it uses a key word, you will beat it up badly. So, as you get stronger, the Voice will get sneakier and attempt to disguise what it is doing. It does this by making a statement of fact followed by silence.

Before you begin Voice Fighting, the Voice would make a typical comment such as, "What a rotten person you are for blowing your assignment like that." Now, with your new skills, you can easily and effectively jump on this kind of statement and stomp the Voice out of your life. So now the Voice will trick you by camouflaging the key word. It will do this by using three different methods: *statements*, *demands*, and *questions*. Your job will be to interrogate the Voice so that you can uncover the key word.

Statements

If the Voice made the statement "You really blew it that time," you would have to *guess* the key word. It could be any one of the six. For instance, the Voice could mean that you couldn't *stand* "blowing it." Or it might be implying that you "*shouldn't* have blown it." Or it might want you to think someone else was *awful* for making you blow it. Or it might be hinting that a *tragedy* would occur if you were to blow it again. Or it might be insinuating that how you feel after blowing it is really *dangerous*.

In other words, any key word can underlie a statement of fact. It is your job to discover which key word. If you merely guess, you only have a one-in-six chance of getting the right one. So, when the Voice makes a statement, you must do something to find out which key word is behind the statement. You have to play detective in order to collect the information you need to fight back.

The only effective way to interrogate the Voice is to ask it a question every time it makes a statement. This question must always take the following form: "So what if . . . ?" By doing this, you ferret out what key word the Voice is playing—which means that you will then have the information you need to clobber it.

Consider the following dialogue:

Voice	Victim
Well, you sure blew it that time.	So what if I blew it?
What do you mean, so what if? Only an idiot would do something like that.	So what if I'm an idiot?
Only worthless people are idiots.	Aha! I caught you using the key word Worthless [me].

Now that this person has found the key word, they would go to the page in their Voice Fighting Kit with the key word Worthless [me] and walk themselves through the Basic Voice Fighting Response.

When using this interrogation technique, many beginners make three common errors:

☐ "I can't just say 'so what if', because this is not a trivial matter."

☐ "I don't believe myself when I say 'So what if . . . ?' "

☐ After saying "so what if" a couple of times, it is easy to give in to the Voice and use old ways of responding.

The first error occurs because of confusion over the meaning of "So what if . . . ?" This response to the Voice is not supposed to mean that you don't care or that what you say is not important. Although this is what the phrase means in everyday language, your use of the phrase against the Voice has a very special and different meaning. The phrase, "So what if. . . ?" means "You're talking to me and hiding the key word, Voice. I've decided to come after you and force you to give me the key word."

This is exactly what happens. Every time you use this phrase, the Voice will talk back to you. If you can keep the Voice talking long enough, you will eventually find the key word. Once you have the key word, you can pummel the Voice right out of your life.

The second error is the result of not understanding the relationship between statements and belief. The Voice wants you to maintain that you must believe something before you can say it. This, as with most things the Voice says, is totally backwards. The truth of the matter is that belief comes after a statement, not before it. If you say something long enough, you will eventually believe it. In fact, that is exactly the reason you are saying all these new things to the Voice—in order to believe them.

The third error is usually the result of inexperience and will easily be corrected with lots and lots of practice. The Voice will be persistent, and after a couple of attempts to say "So what if . . . ?" you may be tempted to throw in the towel. But you can learn to outlast the Voice. If you can stay with the interrogation until you find the key word, then you will begin to sense a new feeling of power in your struggle against the Voice.

Demands

The second form of camouflage used by the Voice is the demand. You can always spot this because of the sense of urgency in the Voice. Instead of telling you how nice it would feel to binge or avoid food, it will tell you to *Binge now!* or *Leave the table now!* Your best defense against the demand is to ask it another, but different question. When the Voice makes a demand, you say, "Why should I . . . ?" This will often get the Voice to go back to making statements. It really doesn't make any difference what the Voice says next; you will have a proper and powerful response ready and waiting.

Questions

Sometimes the Voice will throw a curve ball by asking a question such as, "Well, what are you going to do about feeling bloated?" This is always a difficult position to be in, because your natural response is to try answering the Voice. Never, repeat *never*, directly answer any question the Voice asks you. Instead, always reply with this formula statement: "It's none of your business!"

To dialogue with the Voice when it is talking to you is to always be doomed to failure. Your purpose in the interrogation process is to put the Voice on the defensive. (If you want to verify this, have a friend role-play the interrogation process while you play the Voice. When you start getting nothing but "So what if . . . ?" "Why should I . . . ?" and "It's none of your business," you will see how frustrating it is for the Voice.) If you begin answering questions from the Voice, it has you right where it wants you. You must interrogate the Voice, not be interrogated by it.

Using the Voice Fighting Decision Tree

To help you sort through your responses to the Voice, look at the Voice Fighting Decision Tree. Notice that there are four—and *only* four—ways of responding to the Voice.

1. You will use your Basic Voice Fighting Response if the Voice is using a key word with you.

2. You will ask a question if the Voice is making a statement.

3. You will ask a different question if the Voice is making a demand.

4. You will make a statement every time the Voice asks you a question.

At the top of the flow chart, you see the question, "What is the Voice saying?" By now you are probably able to identify the Voice's messages easier. Follow the arrow to the left and down and you notice that the first major decision is whether the Voice is using a key word with you or not. If it is, you follow the arrow downward and find out that you need to turn to the page in your Voice Fighting Kit which has the appropriate key word at the top.

Now go back to the box which says, "Can you find a key word?" If the Voice did not use a key word, follow the arrow to the right and answer the next question, "Is it a statement?" If the message is a statement, the prompt immediately under the box tells you what to say to the Voice—"So what if. . . ?"

If the Voice did not use a key word or statement, the next question asks if the Voice has made a demand. If so, the prompt under this box tells you to reply back to the Voice with "Why should I. . . ?"

Finally, if the Voice did not use a key word, make a statement or a demand, then it must be asking you a question (remember, these are the only options). You then vigorously retort, "It's none of your business, Voice!"

You will notice that after each of these replies, the next question asks you if the Voice is still bothering you. If you are lucky and the Voice is silenced, then you get to quit for the moment. This won't happen often, but if it does, enjoy the respite.

If the Voice is still talking to you, then you need to determine if it is repeating itself. If it is saying something new or different, then you follow the arrow all the way back to the top and start over. You will continue going in this cycle until the Voice either shuts up or repeats itself.

When the Voice starts saying the same things over and over, then you will notice in the lower right-hand corner of the flow chart that you use your canned phrase which we talked about earlier in this chapter. You will most likely have to use it more that once, but not more than three times. Then you are finished. You can walk away because you have earned it. Take a mental vacation and enjoy a few moments to yourself with someone who is nice to you.

When you first start out Voice Fighting, you must follow this procedure to the letter. If you try to improvise or ad lib, you will find that the Voice will most certainly defeat you as you get totally confused and disoriented. Later on, you will have this flow chart committed to memory and it will be a new habit for you. At that point you will find that you can shorten the whole process considerably—for the extremely experienced Voice fighter, the whole procedure may take just a few seconds.

Using Your Voice Fighting Kit

When you fight the Voice, you can do so three different ways: mentally, verbally, or in writing. Mental fighting is the most convenient, but the most risky at this point. Since you are merely a beginner at Voice Fighting, the Voice is much too quick for you. It has been tormenting you mentally for many years and is an expert at what it does. Since it can operate at such rapid speed, you are currently no match for fighting the Voice mentally. Remember the Voice's two best weapons? Secrecy and speed are what you need to counteract. You must learn to slow it down. You can do this by talking out loud to the Voice (best not done with others around!). Since you can think at a rate of about 400 words a minute and talk at about 100 words a minute, you can slow the Voice down by a factor of four by fighting it aloud—a considerable improvement for you.

You can slow down the Voice even further by writing down your Voice Fighting responses. You can probably write no faster than 20 words a minute—which means that you can slow down the Voice by a factor of 20. It is as if you have watched a movie at regular speed, then in slow motion, and finally in stop action. The last two speeds would certainly give you more time to think. To fight the Voice on paper is relatively simple. You draw a vertical line down the middle of a sheet of paper. Everything the Voice says goes on the left side, and your responses go on the right side. If the Voice keeps rambling and doesn't let you respond, go ahead and cut it off after a sentence or two. Make your response, then listen some more.

On the next page is an example of written Voice Fighting that was completed by June, a female bulimic in her mid-thirties. Notice that she is careful not to guess at the specific Voice key word before it actually appears on the paper.

By always carrying your Voice Fighting Kit with you, you can be ready to meet the Voice wherever and whenever it wants to give you a hard time. Don't allow the Voice to tell you that you shouldn't have to use your Kit. The Voice will try to get you to fight it from memory or make you ashamed to use your Voice Fighting Kit. This is sheer nonsense. Anything you can do to help you fight the Voice is legitimate.

After you have used your Voice Fighting Kit for several weeks or so, you may want to modify some of the Voice Arguments. In general, you need to always update any tools or techniques you have learned from this book so that they can work better for you.

You will find that there are some places where you will not be able to fight the Voice either in writing or out loud. What you need to do at

Voice

You have to go to a pot-
luck tonight.

There will be a lot of
food there.

There will also be a lot
of desserts.

You always binge on
desserts.

Don't go!

Don't you care if you
eat too many desserts?

If you try to resist binging, you will feel awful.

You won't be able to
stand it.

June

So what if I have to go to
a potluck tonight?

So what if there will be a
lot of food there?

So what if there will be a
lot of desserts?

So what if I *always* binge
on desserts?

Why shouldn't I go?

It's none of your business,
Voice.

So what if I feel awful?

Aha—I caught you.

1. Voice, you're trying to
make me feel helpless.

2. You're trying to make
me run away.

3. You're telling me that I
can't stand seeing desserts
and not eating them.

4. The Truth is I have
been standing it all my
life.

5. I am strong and can
control myself even
around desserts; other
people don't feel helpless
around desserts because
they don't agree with
you, Voice.

that point is to remember the details of what the Voice has said to you. This can best be done by carrying a small notebook or index card with you so that you can make notes to use in fighting the Voice at a later time. When you find yourself in a public place or with friends and all of a sudden the Voice starts to really give you a hard time, you can always excuse yourself, go to the restroom, and either take notes on what the Voice is saying to you or actually fight it for five minutes or so. Having your Voice Fighting Kit at this point is invaluable. This should help you to calm down. In addition to fighting the Voice, you can use your other techniques too. Don't forget your stress reduction techniques of natural breathing, muscle relaxation, and mental imagery.

Voice Fighting Styles

You also have three different Voice Fighting styles available to you: rehearsal, reality, and replay. When you fight the Voice before it attacks you, you are using the rehearsal style of Voice Fighting. Fighting the Voice after the battle is over is called the replay style of fighting. The reality style fights the Voice at the time it is bothering you. Each method can be useful to you.

You will want to use the rehearsal style whenever you anticipate a big event that might act as a Voice Trigger. This style is a very powerful method for dealing with the Voice before it can build up its strength to superhuman levels.

Reality Voice Fighting is important because you can deal with the Voice while it is actually doing a number on you. This is often the most difficult method of Voice Fighting, because you must hear, analyze, and remember to use your Voice Fighting Kit at the very moment when the Voice is shouting at you and distracting you.

Fighting the Voice after it is all over is also important. Even though this style may not be as powerful as the reality style, it does give you a chance to practice and sharpen your skills. It will also help you to be more adept at knowing what to say the next time the Voice comes around with the same message.

Voice Letters

Since you now have the tools to get the Voice out of your life, you are on the brink of a whole new life. You need to let the Voice know this and to tell it how you are going to take charge of your life. To do this, you need to write the Voice a letter. Let all your resentment hang out, show all the toughness and meanness in you. Tell the Voice that you mean business, that you are finally going to take a stand and throw it out of your life. Below are some samples of letters written by other people who have learned how to fight the Voice.

Dear Voice:

This is the letter I'm sure you've been dreading, but here it is! You and I are through. I have packed your bags and they are sitting just outside the front door to my head. I've been waiting around for you to leave with them but you just don't take a hint. So, I'm telling you in plain English—GET OUT!

It doesn't matter how you got inside my mind in the first place, and it doesn't matter why I let you stay there all these years. What really matters is that I have decided to remove you from my head and from my life. You've been of no value to me, *ever*, and I am very excited about the prospect of living without you!

This may seem pretty extreme. Well, I learned to be extreme from you. So, as my final extreme act, I am telling you to BE OFF! ! !

Your ex-friend,

Dear Voice,

Thank you for all you've done for me all these years. For ten years you've been disguising yourself as MY conscience. You've got a lot of damn nerve! You told me that I was a complete failure as a person because I had made so many mistakes in my life. I believed you when you told me that making mistakes was terrible and that I was a scum bag. You had me so completely brainwashed that I stopped listening to myself and believing in myself. I had no confidence in my own mind and had lost whatever it was that made me so uniquely me.

I had a joyful spirit in the beginning—you robbed me of that as fast as you possibly could. You wanted me to feel guilty for everyone and everything that was wrong in the world. You wanted me so depressed and miserable that I would have no choice left but to destroy myself. You wanted me so submissive that I would sell my soul in order to have people like me.

And I was so gullible and vulnerable that I let you move in for the slow kill without even realizing what you were doing to me. You were trying to slowly drive me to the brink—trying to make me into a quivering mass of nerves, a person who finally surrendered to you, your lies, and your distorted, sick versions of reality.

Well, guess what, sucker. Knowledge is power and I'm acquiring lots of knowledge about you and your little games. Right now I'm in boot camp. For eight more weeks I'll be taught the strategy and maneuvers I need to fight you. I will learn all your weaknesses and disguises so that I can defeat you and put you out of my life forever. I need an enormous amount of weaponry to fight you and I realize that now. I must admit, you were a formidable opponent...an enemy worth destroying.

You're going to have a vicious opponent in me because, you see, I haven't been letting myself get angry for years. I've been holding this anger in for a long time, and guess who's going to see the brunt of it...you!

I'm fighting for my life. I feel I have a contribution to make on this planet and you aren't going to take that away from me anymore! I'm taking over control now and phasing you out. ADIOS, SUCKER! ! !

You ain't seen the last of me yet, Jerk!

Voice Picture

Some people have found it useful to try to visualize what the Voice looks like to them. Whether you have any artistic talent or not, you may want to do this. It may be something mean and ugly or it may be something very wispy and vague. Or it may be something very attractive and seductive. One of my male clients drew two pictures: one very evil looking and one very friendly. He said that the friendly one was what the Voice looked like when it was trying to set him up for the evil one. However you see your Voice, go ahead and draw it in your notebook.

Typical Voice Fighting Errors

1. **Mislabelling your emotion.** You must be certain that you have identified the correct destructive emotion. If you assume that the Voice is giving you one message when it is actually using another, you can fight all day and not make any progress. This error is very common to the beginner. You can tell when this is happening by comparing your results to your effort. If you are spending considerable time and energy in fighting the Voice but making no gains, the chances are that you are not fighting the right message.

2. **Stopping interrogation prematurely.** When you first begin Voice Fighting, you may find it difficult to continue saying "So what if..." to the Voice. Often, after several attempts at this, the Voice throws something heavy-duty at you and you buckle under by trying to answer back or worse yet agreeing with what it is saying. By writing down what you are saying, you will find it easier to go back over the fight and see if

you are giving in too soon. Remember that you can say "So what if . . . ?" for hours, days, or weeks if you have to.

3. **Getting confused when you win.** Many times a first Voice Fighter will do much better than ever expected. If the Voice shuts up after a few volleys, you can be in for quite a shock. Many people get flustered at this point, because it is such a new experience. Some individuals even become upset because they don't know what to do next. What you do next is to enjoy yourself. Take advantage of the Voice's absence to have some fun.

4. **Moving too quickly against the Voice.** At this point in your Voice Fighting you need to perfect your defensive tactics. Later on, you will learn to take the offensive against the Voice. To play good defense, you must know your opponent and wait for him to commit himself. Let the Voice lead, and then when you see what is happening, pounce!

5. **Shortcutting your Basic Voice Fighting Response.** Impatience can get you into a real jam. The Voice will tell you not to waste your time going through all five steps. As usual, it is lying to you. If you use just the arguments, you will diminish the impact of your Voice Fighting. Always use your Voice Fighting Kit, even if you are sure you have it memorized. Be sure to follow the flow chart exactly as you have it. Later, when you have become an expert, you can take shortcuts and do quite well against the Voice.

6. **Insisting on reasons.** You will defeat your entire purpose if you insist on finding the reasons for your eating disorder. The reasons are unimportant at this time in your life. They merely satisfy your curiosity. Finding reasons can be done after you have become victorious over the Voice.

7. **Memorizing the Voice Fighting Kit.** After you've been using your Kit for several months, the Voice will try to shame you into leaving it behind by telling you that you shouldn't have to rely on a pack of stupid index cards anymore. Of course, if you buy this suggestion, the Voice has a better shot at you when you are stressed and confused.

8. **Mental Voice Fighting.** Although this is the style of fighting you eventually want to become proficient at, the present is too soon to rely on this style to give you much help. The Voice is still too fast for you. You must slow it down, which is done using the other two fighting methods: verbal and written.

9. **Relying on Distraction Response.** When you begin to have some victories against the Voice, you begin to have more and more good days. It is very tempting on your good days to completely forget everything that you have learned about the Voice. Your Good-Day Rule is: ON

GOOD DAYS YOU WORK TWICE AS HARD! Remember to schedule in Voice Fighting times every day. If, at the appointed time, the Voice is nowhere to be seen, then use rehearsal fighting or replay fighting.

The rehearsal method is like any athletic practice session. It is to prepare you for the actual contest. You think of something happening in the immediate future that the Voice will use against you. Try to anticipate the games and practice fighting them in advance.

The replay method is like watching a videotape after the big game. It is a means of finding your weaknesses and strengthening them in preparation for the rematch. Practicing past fights can be an excellent means of improving your self-confidence and Voice Fighting ability.

10. **Hearing only one key word.** If you have a persistent Voice, it is possible that one particular key word may overshadow all the others. For example, your Voice may overshadow all the others. For example, your Voice may continually use tragedy or "should" to the exclusion of the other key words. This actually gives you an advantage, because it is easy for you to anticipate the key word and fight back. If this happens to you, you only have to watch out for the emergence of the other games as you gain more power over the main one.

Additional Voice Fighting Tips

Even though you are in Phase III of your Voice Training, you must still continue to use the skills learned in the first two phases. Be sure you keep watching your pronouns and thus refuse to accept responsibility for negative thoughts and statements. Have your support person or therapist contract with you to give you feedback every time he or she hears you use the word "I" with a negative statement.

If you become overwhelmed by the Voice because it caught you by surprise or because it is using all the key words at once, strike back in a methodical way. You can do this by slowly going through your Voice Fighting Kit and considering each destructive emotion one by one. This will often give you the extra help needed to have a successful fight.

Always try to anticipate Voice Triggers—those situations that trigger off the Voice. In Phase V you will be shown how to attack these triggers methodically. But you can begin to attack Voice Triggers even now. Always try to think at least a few hours or days ahead. When you identify a potentially difficult situation, start fighting the Voice immediately by using the rehearsal style. Then, when the actual situation arrives, you will be more prepared. You may even surprise yourself by how well you do.

If your Voice Fighting becomes lifeless and you feel as though you are just going through the motions, you may need to tap into your feelings of anger and rage. Many people are so used to being run over by the Voice that they can't see the incredible injustice of being someone's slave. When you stop to think of it, surely you must realize that you have the right to be angry at the Voice for what it has done to you. Inject some of this anger into your Voice Fighting.

Don't become upset by occasional defeats. These happen to everybody. Don't let the Voice trick you by convincing you that you must now be a "perfect" Voice Fighter. Be content with making gradual but uneven progress over the next several months. The speed of your progress is not as important as the direction.

Your Voice Fighting skills are preparing you for the big event in Phase V—Voice Provocation. So, in a sense, you are in training. As with other kinds of training, it may be appropriate at times to skip a training session if you are feeling ill or fatigued. Better not to fight now and do well the next day than to make a feeble attempt, lose, and become discouraged. If you aren't feeling strong, check your nutrition, exercise, and sleep patterns.

Some people are hesitant about using their Voice Fighting Kit in public because of what other people might say to them. This is actually an easy problem to solve. Usually you can conceal what you are doing. If you are in a restaurant or at someone's house, you can always excuse yourself, go to the restroom, and fight the Voice. If someone sees you with your Kit or with your notebook and asks what you are doing, you can use several canned responses:

- "I'm taking a class on personal growth and these are some notes."
- "I've been reading a book on learning to control emotions."
- "I'm practicing improving the quality of my life."

Usually the person will either drop the subject or reply by sharing some personal things in their life. If the person shares personal concerns with you, you can choose whether to tell the person more about what you are doing.

In summary, then, you need to be flexible in Voice Fighting. If, during the course of using the Basic Voice Fighting Response, the Voice starts bringing up the same old garbage you've already dealt with, stop using the Disagreement Response and switch to Recitation. Do this by reciting your canned response, which tells the Voice what you want it to do or where you want it to go. And don't tell it to go to Hawaii—direct it to a much warmer place! If the Voice keeps hassling you, merely repeat what you just said. In fact, repeat it exactly as you just said it. The reason this

technique is called the "broken record" is because that is exactly the way you want to sound. When you have recited your canned phrase three times, stop using Recitation and switch to Distraction. In other words, after you have gotten this far, if the Voice is still bugging you, ignore it! Distract yourself by doing something more pleasant than listening to some twaddle from the Voice. In this way, you can use the Distraction Response to your advantage and go on with your life.

It is essential to remember that if you are not actively fighting the Voice, then you are automatically agreeing with it! You will know this is happening whenever you are experiencing any of the destructive emotions. These emotions are valuable clues that the Voice is stalking you and that you are not fighting back.

You must always anticipate times of stress because these are the times when the Voice will try to regain a foothold in your life. You must be especially cautious when you have had a busy day, when you have been sick, when you are tired, when you have had any biological changes in your body, or when holiday time rolls around. If the Voice tries to come back, one of the first things it will do as soon as you are aware of its presence will be to try to convince you that this time is different—the old techniques of Voice Fighting will not work any more. It will try to get you looking for a magic solution somewhere else other than within yourself. Fortunately, you have all you need to fight the Voice—forever.

Additional Rituals

It is now time to increase the number of morning and evening rituals you have been using each day. You will need to add one for the morning and one for the evening. These new rituals are meant to strengthen your ability to fight the Voice successfully.

Morning Ritual

The reason you have been reading the "Take Time to Live" and the "Rights" statements every morning is to remind yourself how important you are. They have helped you to focus attention on yourself and engage in healthy, selfish behavior. Now it is time to remind yourself every morning of the major obstacle in your way for accomplishing this each day. The Voice Dossier will help you recall the viciousness of the Voice. As long as you can remember that your major barrier to self-improvement is in the Voice, you will have an edge over its influence.

Read the following statements each morning immediately after you read your "Rights." Read them aloud, but not in the mirror.

Voice Dossier

1. The Voice always lies.

2. The Voice completely distorts reality.

3. The Voice hates change.

4. The Voice likes everything in black and white.

5. The Voice wants me to think I am worthless and powerless to change my life.

6. The Voice wants me to obey an unreasonable set of rules.

7. The Voice is repetitious, habitual, and dull!

8. The Voice wants me to judge other people based on their behavior.

9. The Voice will use subtle messages to enslave me.

10. The Voice loves to make me feel obligated by using "should" words.

11. The Voice knows exactly what buttons to push with me.

12. The Voice is malicious, nasty, and sneaky.

13. Everything the Voice says is logically flawed and, at best, a half-truth.

14. Beware of the Voice's observation-assumption trick. For example:

    Observation: Your friend didn't want to come over tonight.
    Assumption: That means you must have done something to hurt her feelings.

15. To agree with the Voice, no matter how reasonable it sounds, is *always* to be defeated.

16. The Voice wants me to get caught in an undertow of emotions, fighting myself around and around in circles.

17. The Voice's best weapons are secrecy and speed; I must expose it and slow it down.

18. The Voice is like the wizard in the *Wizard of Oz*—a tiny, frightened thing trying to get me to believe it is larger than life and quite terrifying.

19. The Voice uses illusion to put fear in the hearts of those who are stronger than it is.

20. The Voice wants to convince me that its cheap tricks are part of the real world.

21. The Voice is a coward. It loves hitting me when I'm down.

22. The Voice's only purpose in life is to survive.

23. If I am not actively fighting the Voice, I am automatically agreeing with its messages.

24. I need to anticipate times of stress, because those are the times when the Voice will try to regain a foothold in my life.

25. Guilt is one of the Voice's tricks to keep me dependent upon the unrealistic expectations of other people.

26. The Voice wants me to be resentful so that I will eventually cut off all human support and caring.

27. The Voice is my worst enemy and wants me to be miserable.

28. The Voice likes to play it safe—the Voice is gutless!

29. The Voice tries to trick me by insisting that a low probability event has a good chance of happening.

30. When I take risks, I challenge the Voice—the Voice wants me to be immobilized with fear.

Evening Ritual

In addition to your other evening rituals, you also need to do a Voice Review. This exercise will last from five to thirty minutes, depending on the type of day you have had. There are two parts to this paper-and-pencil exercise. First, you need to write down what the Voice said to you during the day. This can follow a simple, outline format.

1. You have too many things to do today.

2. You better skip breakfast.

3. You look real ugly in that outfit.

4. You haven't made any progress in therapy, you know.

5. You should stay away from that party tonight.

Although your list may have many more items than this one (this list would indicate a pretty good day), they need not take up more than one line per item, nor do you have to include duplicate items.

When your list is as complete as you can make it, then verbally go through each item and reply to these statements with a good, strong one-liner. If any item happens to explode in your face, then do a full-fledged Voice Fight. Your responses to the list above might go like this:

1. I wouldn't have so many things to do if you would disappear.

2. I'd like to skip on your head.

3. Not as ugly as you're going to look when I get finished with you.

4. I've learned how to nail you and that's enough.

5. I'll decide whether to go or not—it's not your concern.

The Voice Review is intended to clean up the day before retiring and to keep you from dragging any old garbage into the new day. As you make your list, you may also discover some voice messages that you had missed during the day. The more messages you can uncover and mop up, the better your chance will be of beginning a good day and being successful.

Skills Checklist

- ☐ Continue stress reduction exercises
- ☐ Morning rituals (3)
- ☐ Evening rituals (3)
- ☐ Construct Voice Fighting Kit
- ☐ Practice Voice Fighting daily
- ☐ Review this chapter three more times

8

Voice Substitution

To love oneself is the beginning of a life long romance.
—OSCAR WILDE, 1895

The Deadly Diet is death on self-esteem. And a good sense of self-esteem is essential for everyone. It gives us a sense of power in dealing with life. With it we can often go beyond our normal limits and reach a greater potential. The Voice knows that it can keep you shackled by keeping your self-esteem at a continual low ebb. The existence of a healthy self-esteem and the dominating presence of the Voice are mutually exclusive. Both cannot occur at the same time.

Unfortunately, getting rid of the Voice will not automatically improve your self-esteem. In fact, as you get more proficient at Voice Fighting, you may begin to sense an impending vacuum in your life. At this point, the Voice quite commonly reminds people of the Great Abyss.

I first heard of this problem many years ago when I was just beginning to work with eating disorders. As my client was beginning to make substantial progress against the Voice, she became more reluctant to work hard in therapy. When I asked her what was happening, she replied, "I'm scared! The Voice is telling me that if I kick it out of my life there will be nothing left. I feel like I am standing on the edge of a cliff and looking down into a black, bottomless pit." The Voice had been telling this woman that she really didn't want to rid herself of the Voice because there would be nothing left in her life. This is a common ploy that the Voice uses with Deadly Dieters.

For many people, the possibility of finally ridding their lives of something they don't want but have known for a long time feels scary and foreboding. In a sense, this is correct. The Voice has had a grip on your life for so long that it has really become a major part of your existence. If you were to oust the Voice, there would be a mental vacuum. There may be so little of the real you in your thinking that defeating the Voice leaves you feeling empty and alone.

This chapter is designed to fill that void by replacing the space left behind by the Voice with all of the good qualities you potentially have. This chapter is divided into two sections: affirmations and self-exploration. Each of these areas is meant to help you build up your sense of esteem and confidence. As you learn to feel better about yourself, you will be better able to keep the Voice at bay.

But you must keep one thing in mind: Voice Substitution is not a *replacement* for Voice Fighting. It is a *supplement* to Voice Fighting. For many people, this phase is so pleasant and delightful that they forget that the Voice will always try to wiggle its way back. Should it attempt to do so, you must temporarily halt your work in this phase and proceed to fight any attempt by the voice to take over your life. Then, when you have gotten rid of the Voice's presence, you can return to this phase.

This is a critical phase, because when people have experienced some success with the Voice and are enjoying the fruit of their labors, they tend to forget what it was that made them successful. Forgetting about the Voice and resting on the initial success is called the *plateau effect*. Most people who plateau at this point eventually find that the plateau slopes backward. The rude awakening comes when the individual has a setback.

Setbacks are fairly common, so you should not be surprised if and when you have one. They tend to occur soon after a series of good days. They often come as a shock, because you have forgotten to even think of what the Voice can do to you. You will learn more about dealing with setbacks in chapter ten.

To either forestall or lessen the impact of setbacks, you need to be aware of the Voice even on your "good days." When you are having good days it is easy to kick back and enjoy your new-found freedom. If you fail to be aware of the Voice trying to come back, your good days will not last long. Therefore it is of the utmost importance to follow the Good-Day Rule: ON GOOD DAYS YOU WORK TWICE AS HARD.

The work you need to do on your good days is to nurture your sense of worth. When the Voice is more or less leaving you alone, take that time to discover your positive, constructive qualities

Affirmations

Affirmations are a technique you can use to strengthen your self-confidence and increase your personal power. The definition of an affirmation is: *A strong, positive statement about yourself that you do not believe.* That's right! The more you "disbelieve" something about yourself, the better its potential as an affirmation. For example, if you were to tell yourself that you had beautiful red hair, a fact you already knew, this would be a fairly worthless affirmation. However, if you had a hard time believing that you were "wonderful, delightful, and special," then this phrase would make a marvelous affirmation.

Affirmations are meant to serve two purposes. First of all, they fill the vacancy left by the Voice. Second, affirmations serve as self-fulfilling prophesies. We all know that if we hear something long enough we tend to believe it. Affirmations use this observation to your advantage. It is a form of reprogramming your mental state with healthy, positive awareness about yourself.

Affirmation Bank

The first thing you need to do is to develop a repository of strong, positive sayings. Then you can start off each day by picking an affirmation to take with you for that day. If you have a ready list of fifty or so affirmations, you will be able to save time rather than having to devise your daily affirmation from scratch. Listed below are some sample affirmations.

- I can gain weight and still love myself.
- I can use more effective methods of weight control other than binging and purging.
- I can live without hiding behind my Deadly Diet.
- I can gain weight and self-confidence at the same time.
- I am able to completely alter my past routines and rituals.
- I am highly pleasing to myself.
- I am learning to love myself more every day.
- No matter what happens, I can control my fears and doubts.
- I do not need the approval of others for my self-esteem.
- I respect my own uniqueness.
- I like myself even if others are not present.
- I can now practice being good to myself.
- I deserve to be happy.

- I have the ability to rejoice in the happiness of others.
- My self-esteem is not related to my capacity to please others.
- I can draw to me the friends and loved ones I want.
- I know that I don't have to seek absolute perfection in everything I do.
- I feel secure in my own self-worth, individuality, and sense of belonging.
- I have a positive energy within me that draws others to me.
- I am a very positive, sincere, and strong person.
- I can accept pressure and rejection from others.
- I realize that solitude is the opportunity to develop my self-esteem.
- I accept myself—the whole package that is me.
- Even though I have faults and make mistakes, I still love me.
- Since there is no one exactly like me, I am a very interesting person.
- I am a good person and can look for the good in other people.
- Even though I may not like what I do, I still like who I am.
- I am not what I think I am—but what I think, I am.
- I have many talents, skills, and other good qualities to offer.
- I have nothing to be ashamed of.
- I can now practice being good to myself.

As you think of other affirmations, add them to your list. Each day, as you withdraw an affirmation from your bank, put the date beside it so that you can tell when it was used. This affirmation bank needs to be reviewed and updated once or twice a month. The more each affirmation disagrees with what the Voice has been telling you, the better it will work. When you have deposited at least fifty affirmations, you are ready to continue with this chapter.

An Affirmation a Day Keeps the Voice Away

Once you have developed your list of affirmations, you are ready to begin using them. Every morning when you get up, choose an affirmation by either making one up or withdrawing one from your Affirmation Bank. Pick one that speaks strongly and uniquely to you for that particular day. If you think you'll have trouble remembering your affirmation for the day, write it down on an index card and carry it with you. There are three ways for you to practice your affirmations: mentally, verbally, or graphically.

Mental Affirmations

Mental affirmations are probably the easiest to use because you can be anywhere or in any situation when you practice them. To be effective, however, you need to mentally repeat your affirmation about 1000 times each day. Although this may seem like a lot of effort, it really turns out to be very little time at all. Each affirmation takes no more than two seconds to repeat. If you divide the number of hours the average person is awake each day (about 16 hours), you'll find that you need to think your affirmation 62.5 times each hour in order to do it 1000 times in a day. That means that it will take you no more than 125 seconds or about two minutes each hour. If you can remember to mentally repeat your daily affirmation for two minutes each hour in a day, you will have said it at least 1000 times.

This use of affirmations could be called the Steam Roller Technique. True, it is dull and boring, but the repetitious use of the same affirmation over and over and over again will begin to burn into your memory the kinds of things that help you take control of your life. After all, this is the very method the Voice has used with you for many years. It kept telling you all sorts of negative, destructive things until you eventually believed them. It is now time to reverse this process by pouring these powerful, positive statements into your brain. Someday you will actually believe them.

Verbal Affirmations

Another way you can make your affirmations work for you is to say them aloud. Saying them aloud has the advantage of increasing your sense of personal power by actually letting you hear the affirmation. Obviously, you will only want to do this when you are alone—in your car or in your house. Our clients have found two methods for doing this that tend to be quite effective. If you can think of other ways to practice verbal affirmations, by all means do so.

The Mirror Technique. Stand in front of a mirror and try to convince the person in the mirror how important it is for that person to believe the affirmation. Point out to the person in the mirror the significance of the affirmation. Really put yourself into this role. Pretend that you are an actress or an actor playing a part, using every available acting trick you can think of in order to convince yourself how wonderful and exciting the affirmation is.

The Cassette Technique. Another way of practicing verbal affirmations is to use a cassette player. Go to a store specializing in electronic or audio equipment and purchase a "closed loop cassette." A closed loop cassette looks like any other cassette except that it works differently—there is no beginning and there is no end. It just keeps going around and around, constantly repeating whatever is on the tape. You may find different types, such as 30-second, 60-second, or 90-second cassettes. To use this technique, get yourself a 30-second closed loop cassette. Every morning take just a few minutes to record your affirmation on it. Continue recording the affirmation for 30 seconds. Carry the cassette with you during the day. When you are in your car, rather than listening to music and distracting yourself, slip this cassette into the tape player and listen to it as it speaks back to you over and over and over.

Some people think this is what is called "subliminal motivation." It is not. It is nothing more than brute force repetition. (Most of the competent research on subliminal motivation shows that it doesn't work.)

If you record the tape yourself, you may feel uncomfortable hearing your own voice. Very few people enjoy hearing the sound of their own voice for the first time. You probably will be no exception, but time will take care of this difficulty.

Once again, if you can think of other techniques that will enhance your verbal affirmation, do not hesitate to use them. Anything that works is okay. In fact, if you come up with something that works well for you, I would appreciate if you wrote to me in care of the address in the back of the book so that I can pass on your good idea to others.

Written Affirmations

The method of written affirmations is probably the most powerful method of the three. It is also the most cumbersome. This method will take from one to two hours to complete. To use written affirmations, you will need a piece of paper with three columns drawn on it. By looking at the sample below you can see how to set it up.

Affirmation	Voice Response	Your Response

Notice that each column is labelled from left to right, AFFIRMA-TION, VOICE, RESPONSE. You write your affirmation in the left-hand column using the formula, "I, [name], [affirmation]." When you do this, the odds are very high that the Voice will make some type of response to you. Write its response in the middle column. Then reply in the last column with a snappy comeback. Your response does not have to follow the BVFR nor the interrogation techniques you learned in the last chapter. Remember, you are not Voice Fighting when you use this method of written affirmations. You are merely responding to a dumb comment from a weakened Voice trying its feeble best to rattle you.

When you have completed these three columns, you do it all over again by writing the affirmation *in exactly the same way* in column one. The Voice will probably say something different this time. Write it down.

Give another response. Do this twenty times. Look at the illustration below and you will see a sample of how this is done.

When you have completed this set of twenty affirmations, do another set of twenty. This time, change the formula slightly by changing the pronoun "I" to the pronoun "you." Once again, look at the sample illustration. Finally, after you have done twenty "you affirmations," change the pronoun from "you" to "she" or "he" (whichever is appropriate). Refer to the sample to see what this looks like.

Affirmation	Voice Response	Your Response
1. I, Jane Doe, am making very positive changes in my lifestyle.	Oh, sure you are. Any changes you make will be negative ones.	I don't have to listen to you, because I'm in charge of my own life.
2. I, Jane Doe, am making very positive changes in my lifestyle.	You're too helpless to do any good for yourself!	If you think I'm going to buy into that nonsense, you're nuts!!
3. etc.		
1. You, Jane Doe, are making very positive changes in your lifestyle.	The only thing you're going to do is fail—with a splash.	I'm succeeding— you're going to take a hike.
2. You, Jane Doe, are making very positive changes in your lifestyle.	You should have called your mother this morning—she's going to be awfully hurt.	Stop trying to change the subject and make me feel guilty—we'll talk about my mother later.
3. etc.		
1. She, Jane Doe, is making very positive changes in her lifestyle.	She's a no-good nerd.	Bug off!! I don't need your stupid comments anymore.
2. She, Jane Doe, is making very positive changes in her lifestyle.	What are you doing this stupid writing for? You know it doesn't do any good.	Listen, Voice. I'll do anything to get rid of you even if it is stupid.
3. etc.		

You will find this writing affirmation technique very powerful—and very laborious. It has maximum power if you can complete all sixty affirmations in one sitting. If you can't do this, then the next best thing is to complete the affirmations in three sittings. Try doing the first twenty in the morning, the second twenty in the afternoon, and the third twenty in the evening.

Do a set of written affirmations for about a month. Use a new affirmation each day. Use it mentally, verbally, and graphically each day.

After you have used daily affirmations for a month, you'll no longer need to do them every day. Instead, use them when you are having a "good day." Each day of your life, for at least several years, you need to either be fighting the Voice or using affirmations. Or you may need to do both many times in the same day.

Self-Exploration

As a Deadly Dieter, you may have allowed the Voice to suppress the real person inside so much that you don't even know who you are. And now that the Voice has begun to leave your life, you may find it difficult to fully appreciate the joy of being human. In her book, *How to Stop Playing the Weighting Game*, Gloria Arenson has supplied the reader with a wealth of exercises to help build self-esteem and acceptance. The following exercises are adapted from this helpful book and will assist you in exploring an assortment of exciting dimensions in your existence.

An inability to value the attributes that make you unique is part of the dead-end nature of the Deadly Diet. If someone were to ask you, "Who are you?" you might be at a loss. What would you say? Now that the Voice is beginning to recede from your life, it is time for you to discover whether or not you are who you think you are. A valuable clue to who you are can be obtained by comparing what you tell yourself with what your loved ones say about you. You can also find valuable information about yourself by listening to what friends, neighbors, or co-workers say about you.

Begin by listing the first ten words or phrases that come to your mind in answer to the question WHO AM I?

1.

2.

3.

4.

5.

6.

7.

8.

9.

10.

Put a happy face next to each description of yourself which is positive OR realistic. Put a sad fact next to each description that probably comes from the Voice. Now answer the following questions

1. Do I have more positive descriptions than negative ones?

2. How would I have completed this list prior to reading this book and learning to defeat the Voice?

3. What can I do to change the "sad face" descriptions to more positive or realistic ones?

Blessings

As a typical Deadly Dieter, you may find it quite easy to praise others but exceedingly difficult to do the same for yourself. To show you this contrast, I want you to pretend that someone you know has just had a baby. You are visiting this family and are being given the chance to see the baby for the first time. As you look at the newborn, you are overcome with emotion for this lovely creature, who has an entire life ahead of her. Think of what you would like to say to this infant. Think about the tremendous wealth of experience awaiting her. As you think about this, write your good wishes and blessings below by completing the following phrases.

You deserve . . .
You are . . .
You can be . . .
You can do . . .
It's okay to . . .
I wish you . . .
You will . . .
You need to . . .

If you can think of any other blessings to bestow on this baby, feel free to add them to the list. When you have given your best to this child, set aside some time to be alone. Find a mirror and read each of the blessings you gave the child. Use a loving and accepting tone of voice. Precede each blessing with your name. In other words, give yourself the same blessing you just composed for the baby.

When you have completed this little exercise, write about this experience in your notebook. How did these self-blessings make you feel?

What was the Voice telling you? Is it now possible for you to begin to accept these blessings? Are you any less important than the baby?

You have probably already guessed that these blessings look vaguely like affirmations. You might do well to add them to your Affirmation Bank—especially the blessings that really arouse the Voice.

Body Acceptance

Philosophers have told us for many years that we are more than just our bodies. And most of us are aware of something more to our lives than just an outer garment of skin. Yet so many Deadly Dieters have come to believe that the most important thing in the world is their body. I even had one person tell me that she would rather be thin and unhappy than fat and happy. This distorted over-emphasis on how we look is directly related to the bombardment of advertising all of us are exposed to every day. If you watch TV, read newspapers or magazines, or listen to radio, you are constantly being told that your body is the secret to happiness and a long life. As a Deadly Dieter, you probably let the scale or the mirror tell you whether or not you are lovable.

Do you remember when you were a child? How did your looks differ from what they are today? What are the similarities? Many people are unrecognizable from pictures of their childhood. And yet they are the same person. As your body kept changing from childhood to adulthood, you went through many metamorphoses. But as the parts of your body grew and changed shape, you still remained the same person. As the cells in your body died and others took their place, you still remained the same person. Although your body is not permanent, you are!

Because we all have the possibility of making minor adjustments to the way we look, many people spend considerable time and money in fine-tuning their body. Millions of dollars are spent each year to change muscle tone, lose weight, change hair styles and color, and reshape facial structures. These things are the variables. Things that are essentially unchangeable are height, bone structure, and certain proportions. Do any of these permanent items make you hate yourself—even though you can't change them?

When scientists began studying eating disorders, their first discovery was the Deadly Dieter's distorted sense of body image. Even though the person fell far below anybody's standard of weight, she still perceived herself as "fat."

Maybe it is now time for you to begin seeing yourself as you really are. Take a good look in the mirror. Take off your clothes and look yourself over. As you scan your body, write down in your notebook exactly what you see. Make sure that what you write down is what someone else would also see. Don't let the Voice tell you what you see—let your own eyes discover what is there.

One Deadly Dieter discovered that her face was not particularly pretty—with the exception of her eyes. People kept commenting to her about her dark, deep-set eyes. After writing down what she saw in the mirror, the Voice made some nasty comments about her face. Her reply was, "Maybe so, Voice, but what a gorgeous set of eyes." Like most people, you will have to find what you like about yourself and build on those qualities. Maybe you will have to begin by liking your toes, hair, fingernails, mouth, or calves.

After having discovered the parts of your body you enjoy, write down the things you don't like about your body. Next to each item, indicate whether or not it is possible to change that item.

The Real You

Archeologists are people who study the past. They spend much of their time digging in the earth for treasures now lost and buried. When valuable artifacts are finally discovered, it takes an experienced eye to see through the soiled encrustation of the ages. Once the article has been cleaned, the beauty is often stunning. The Voice has made you a relic of your past. When you clean up your life by ridding yourself of the Voice, you too will be aware of the shining beauty of the real you.

The exercises in this chapter are a means of dusting yourself off. They will bring out what has been hidden from you all this time. To begin, you need to enumerate all the qualities in yourself that are positive. Put down everything you like about yourself. There is nothing too small for your list.

To get you started, it may be helpful to discover how you are similar to those you admire. Think of someone from your childhood whom you loved and admired. What was their name? What was their relationship to you? Write in your notebook all the things about this person that were special.

Next think of someone famous in fact or fiction whom you admire. Who is this person? What is or was special about this person?

Finally, identify someone you love today. Write down his or her name and special qualities in your notebook. When you have listed all the positive qualities of these three people, ask yourself how you compare to each of them. Describe in detail the qualities and talents you have in common with the person you chose from your childhood Then do the same for each of the other two. When you have finished, make a list that includes all of your positive qualities that are similar to those of these three people.

This list can act as an insurance policy for defeat. As a Deadly Dieter, one of your worst times is when you give in to the Voice. When this happens, the Voice further compounds your defeat by telling you that you are no good and a complete failure. This list of positive qualities will help to cushion your setback. Setbacks are normal and need to be seen in the light of human nature. Even when you have setbacks, it doesn't mean you are not a good friend, compassionate, intelligent, faithful, honest, loving, talented, creative, and so on. It only means you blew it. Big deal! Remember, your worth is not equal to your behavior.

The Deadly Dieter Double Standard

As a typical Deadly Dieter, you probably find it quite easy to make allowances for the shortcomings of other people. However, it is very difficult to give yourself the same benefit. You judge yourself with a different set of standards than you use on other people.

Have you ever had the experience of not liking someone because they didn't make a good first impression? Sometimes the first impression fades as you get to know that person.

Gloria Arenson tells of working as a volunteer during an election many years ago. One day she was introduced to an elderly woman. When she reported the incident to her friends she did not say, "I met an old, wrinkled, buck-toothed lady today." She said, "I met Eleanor Roosevelt, and she shook my hand!" Mrs. Roosevelt was more than what she looked like on the outside—and the same goes for you. No matter how you look, you can be worthwhile, lovable, and happy. You, as a person, will always remain special and wonderful.

To help you rid yourself of the double standard, answer the following questions.

1. Write down the name of a person you cared about who was:
   - old
   - handicapped
   - ugly
   - fat

   What difference did these outward characteristics make in your friendship?

   If the situation were reversed, would the other person still have cared for you?

2. Write down the name of someone you love today who is not overweight.

   Now imagine how this person would look if he/she gained 50 pounds. Would you stop loving him or her?

   What is it that you really love about this person?

3. Write down the name of someone who loves or cares deeply about you today.

If you became ill, would that person stop loving you?

If you were to become handicapped, would that person stop loving you?

What is it about you that this person loves?

Skills Checklist

☐ Continue stress reduction exercises—recall, eyes open, noise

☐ Morning rituals (4)

☐ Evening rituals (4)

☐ Complete mental, verbal, and written affirmations daily

☐ Continue Voice Fighting during bad times

9

Voice Provocation

Not everything that is faced can be changed,
but nothing can be changed until it is faced.

—JAMES BALDWIN

In chapter one you learned that the real issue in the Deadly Diet is not eating, but rather the loss of control. This loss of control is directly related to how much influence the Voice has in your life. Now that you know how to remove the Voice and substitute something better—namely, yourself—it is time to begin changing your entire negative lifestyle.

The Goal of Voice Provocation

A steady diet of Voice Provocation will keep you from being influenced by the plateau effect. The plateau effect becomes a problem for many people at this point in their progress because pain has been such an excellent motivator; the absence of pain can sometimes completely stop any forward momentum. If this has happened to you, you may be tempted to ease up on using some of the skills that you have learned so far. This dangerous decision could invite the Voice to come back and re-take control of your life, resulting in the loss of many of the gains you have made.

Voice Provocation can best be thought of as switching from playing a defensive game to playing an offensive game. Up to this point, you have been learning a strong defensive game. You have learned how to effectively counter many of the attacks by the Voice. As you get stronger and stronger, the Voice is less willing to attack you directly. So it goes into hiding and attacks you when you are not ready—when you are fatigued, sick, or stressed. Instead of conventional warfare, the Voice is now waging guerrilla warfare. You may go days or even weeks without any serious Voice problems. Then all of a sudden the Voice will attack you "from out of the blue." It would be much better if you could learn to flush the Voice from its hiding place before it attacks. This can be done by using Voice Provocation.

By switching from a defensive strategy to an offensive one, you can put all of your strength into striking first. In other words, you need to find the Voice before it finds you. This is often a scary prospect. You may wonder, "Why not leave well enough alone? Why provoke the Voice just when it is starting to leave me alone?" Voice Provocation is absolutely necessary because you need to prove to yourself (and to the Voice) that you really can control your life.

This is not an easy skill to learn. After all, the Voice does not want you to bring it back out into the open. You know by now that one of its best weapons is secrecy. It can gain the upper hand by staying hidden and then attacking when you least expect it. Your task, then, is to force it into the open; you want to drive it out of its hiding place.

You can do this in one of two ways. The Control Cycle showed you two types of Voice Triggers: the situation and your own behavior. So all you have to do to provoke the Voice is something that the Voice has been telling you not to do. For example, you could eat some forbidden food, eat "too much" food, weigh yourself, or even exercise less.

Various situations can also trigger the Voice—having someone comment on your weight, finding that a certain article of clothing is tight, or feeling stressed. Your assignment in this chapter will be to identify Voice Triggers, use them to bring the Voice out of hiding, and then show it who is boss by stomping on it.

You will divide these triggers into two lists: a list of food-related triggers and a list of nonfood-related triggers. These triggers will be ranked from the most intense to the least intense on a scale of one to ten. You will begin Voice Provocation by first dealing with the least intense triggers. After you have built up your confidence with these lesser triggers, you will then go after bigger game until you eventually are ready and strong enough to neutralize the most difficult triggers in your life.

To really liberate yourself from the Voice and to put yourself in complete charge of your own life, you must begin to provoke the Voice on a regular basis. It needs to have top priority in your Daily Schedule. But because of a natural tendency to avoid difficult situations and behaviors, this portion of the Voice Training is the downfall of many Deadly Dieters. Unless you vigorously and actively engage in Voice Provocation on a regular basis, you will continue to be at the mercy of the Voice—it will always put limitations on your life.

Constructing Your Trigger Hierarchy

Your first step in Voice Provocation is to identify the Voice Triggers in your life. To do this, complete the following Voice Trigger Inventory. This Inventory contains a wide range of Voice Triggers, but it may miss many of the significant ones in your life. So when you have completed the Inventory, add as many of your own triggers as you can think of. Check off those triggers that tend to get the Voice to bother you. Be sure to also identify any infrequent triggers.

Voice Trigger Inventory

- [ ] Being in a strange place
- [ ] Doing something embarrassing
- [ ] Loud voices
- [ ] Being left out of a group
- [ ] Speaking in public
- [ ] Making a decision
- [ ] Entering a room where people are already seated
- [ ] Seeing yourself in a mirror
- [ ] Dentists
- [ ] People telling you you're fat
- [ ] Failure
- [ ] Having someone look at you "funny"
- [ ] Receiving injections
- [ ] Feeling full (bloated)
- [ ] Strangers
- [ ] Having a missed heartbeat
- [ ] Feeling angry
- [ ] Eating "junk food"
- [ ] Being teased
- [ ] Crowds
- [ ] Being accused of something
- [ ] Group pressure
- [ ] Being alone
- [ ] Seeing fat people
- [ ] Someone telling you that you have put on a little weight
- [ ] Being watched working
- [ ] Stepping on a scale
- [ ] Rejection
- [ ] Making a mistake
- [ ] Doing "something stupid" in public
- [ ] Compliments
- [ ] Diagreements
- [ ] Angry people
- [ ] Exercising your rights
- [ ] Watching other people eat
- [ ] Not getting all your work done

- ☐ People in authority
- ☐ Sudden noises
- ☐ Introducing yourself to a stranger
- ☐ Expressing your feelings
- ☐ Buying clothes
- ☐ Asking permission
- ☐ Being around people who "have it all together"
- ☐ Doing something sloppy
- ☐ Wasting time
- ☐ People telling you that you look thin
- ☐ Hunger
- ☐ Tired
- ☐ Not getting enough exercise
- ☐ Having someone persuade you to do something you don't want to do

Voice Box

Your next step is to make a Voice Box. For this you will need a recipe box, a stack of index cards, and eleven tabbed dividers that will fit into the recipe box. Ten of the dividers will be numbered from one to ten. The last divider, labelled "R.I.P.," will be used for those triggers that no longer activate the Voice. Put this divider behind all the others in your Voice Box.

Begin to construct hierarchies, one trigger at a time. You will need a fairly large workspace to do this. Choose an item from the inventory and try to imagine the worst possible example of this trigger. If you have chosen stepping on a scale as a trigger, gaining five pounds may be the worst example you can think of. Put this example on an index card and give it a rating between one and ten. A ranking of one would indicate a mildly irritating trigger; ten would be a trigger that brings on a panic attack. Be careful about calling any trigger a ten. There is nothing worse than a ten, and true tens are fairly rare. If you don't have panic attacks, none of your triggers should be ranked as a ten, no matter how awful they feel.

If you decided that stepping on a scale and seeing yourself five pounds heavier was a seven, then put a seven in the upper right-hand corner of the index card. Place a blank card underneath this card and try to imagine a related trigger that would be less intense. Perhaps seeing that you had gained four pounds might be a six. Put this trigger, "standing on a scale and seeing myself four pounds heavier," at the top of this blank index card with the number six in the upper right-hand corner. Another blank card underneath this one would be used to identify a five trigger and so on until you reached a trigger with a rating of one. When you finish constructing a hierarchy for stepping on a scale, you will have a column of seven cards in front of you, each with a separate but related trigger ranked from one to seven. You would then put these seven cards into the Voice Box behind the appropriate index dividers. The one trigger would go behind the number one divider, the two trigger behind the number two divider, and so on.

Another person might construct a different hierarchy from the trigger "standing on a scale." This person might find that just standing on a scale and looking at her weight, regardless of how much it is, is a six trigger. Standing on the scale but not looking at the weight might be a five. Watching someone else standing on a scale might be a four; standing next to the scale might be a three; looking at the scale might be a two; just having the scale in the house could be a one. You can see that after giving a rating to the worst example, your chosen trigger is then used to create a series of lesser triggers that are related to the worst trigger. Each of these steps allows you to gradually work toward overcoming the worst example of the trigger. It is this series of examples, graduated from one to a higher number, which is called a *hierarchy*. The number of steps in the hierarchy will equal the number you have assigned to the worst example of the trigger. When you have finished a hierarchy, place the index cards for each step into the Voice Box. Then, choose another trigger from your inventory and make another hierarchy.

If you have difficulty thinking of smaller, related steps for your hierarchy, it often helps to identify the different components or variables that make up your worst example. For example, Judy had picked "seeing myself in the mirror" as an event that easily triggered the Voice. After some thought, she realized that it was the degree to which she saw the shape of her body that decided how strong the trigger was. Obviously this meant that the strongest example of this trigger was seeing herself in the nude. She put this specific trigger example on an index card. On the ten-point scale of Voice Trigger intensity, she decided that this trigger deserved about a six. She placed this card on a table and made a column of five more cards directly underneath. Each card in this column was given another trigger slightly less intense than the one above it. She did this by gradually adding clothing to obscure the details of her body. When Judy had finished her hierarchy, it looked like this:

6 - seeing myself in the nude
5 - seeing myself in a bikini
4 - seeing myself in my aerobic outfit
3 - seeing myself in tight-fitting jeans and a T-shirt
2 - seeing myself in loose-fitting clothes
1 - seeing myself all dressed up

If you have decided that eating 1800 calories in one day—without purging—is a ten, put this trigger card, "eating 1800 calories," on the table. Since you rated it a ten, put nine blank cards in a column underneath this card.

Next, try to imagine an activity similar to "eating 1800 calories," but not quite as powerful. In this case, maybe eating 1700 calories would be a strong trigger, but not as strong as "eating 1800 calories." Write "eating 1700 calories" on the card beneath the "eating 1800 calories" card. Rank this card as a nine.

Use the same procedure for the third card from the top. This might be labelled "eating 1600 calories" and given an eight. Continue until you have completed the bottom card. In this case it would be "eating 900 calories," and the rating would be a one. When you have completed all of the cards in the column, place each card behind the appropriate numbered divider in your Voice Box.

Your next trigger might be "eating in restaurants." Since this example is more difficult to assign specific numbers for, you would need to identify all of the possible variables for eating in restaurants. The variables might be:

a. eating in a familiar or unfamiliar restaurant
b. eating with a group of people or just one other person
c. eating with someone I know or a stranger

You might decide that the worst possible example of this situation would be eating dinner at an unknown restaurant with one person who was a stranger. This trigger might be so stressful that a rating of eight would be appropriate. You would then take eight blank cards and make your hierarchy. Here is an example of what this hierarchy might look like.

8 - eating dinner at an unknown restaurant with a person I don't know
7 - eating dinner at an unknown restaurant with a group of strangers
6 - eating dinner at an unknown restaurant with a group of friends
5 - eating dinner at an unknown restaurant with a single friend
4 - eating dinner at a familiar restaurant with a stranger
3 - eating dinner at a familiar restaurant with a group of strangers
2 - eating dinner at a familiar restaurant with a group of friends
1 - eating dinner at a familiar restaurant with a friend

You must remember this is only an example. Your own hierarchy for restaurant-eating might be considerably different, depending on the variables that were important to you.

Provoking the Voice

Impediments

Many Deadly Dieters are quite reluctant to make a strong commitment to Voice Provocation. Life without the Voice feels so good that it doesn't make sense to needlessly stir up the Voice. Who in their right mind wants to poke a stick into a hornet's nest? The person who wants mastery over the hornets, that's who. And to prove your mastery over the Voice, provoking it is essential.

Perhaps you would rather not provoke the Voice because you don't "feel" strong enough to do it yet. If this is true, then continue Voice Fighting and Voice Substitution until you really are stronger. But don't trust your feelings! You can gauge your strength by the entries in your Success Diary.

And don't let the Voice trick you into thinking you are not ready for this last phase of Voice Training when in fact you really are. The Voice will want you to focus on the highest step of your hierarchies. This is silly! You won't even begin to work on these items until you have successfully completed all the lower items. You will begin at such an easy level that your success will be guaranteed.

Even at this stage, you may still be unsure of what life will be like without the Voice. Believe me, it will be light-years ahead of having the Voice as your constant companion. One of the last scams the Voice will try on you will be to nag you about how lonely you will be without its presence. Yes, you will feel an emptiness and some discomfort without the familiarity of the Voice. But you will soon readjust and get to the place where your self will be more familiar than the Voice.

Begin Provocation Gradually

When your Voice Box contains the hierarchies for all of your triggers, you are ready to begin Voice Provocation. You will begin by using the level one triggers in slot number one to provoke the Voice. Your intention is to make the Voice molest you so that you can beat it back down. The reason for beginning with the level one triggers is to ensure your success. Although this approach may seem incredibly slow, it also is a way to structure your success. When you have mastered the level one triggers, the level two triggers will not be very difficult. Likewise, when you have mastered the level nine triggers, the level ten triggers will be a minor jump.

How long it will take you to reach level ten is entirely up to you. It is better to go too slow than too fast. Remember, your goal is not to reach level ten as soon as you can, but rather to defeat the Voice all along the way. Many people think the goal is to *engage* in level ten triggers. This is a dangerous misconception. Your goal is to defeat the Voice in level ten trigger situations.

It is quite possible that you will be working on your Voice Box for several years or even for the rest of your life. You can see the advantage of doing this. Whenever a difficult situation arises in your life from now on, you can create a hierarchy for it and gradually work on defeating the Voice. You now have a technique for reducing monumental events down into a series of smaller, more manageable events. It is like stuffing an evil genie back into its bottle.

Since you will start Voice Provocation with such low intensity triggers, the provocation will be minor, and your ability to handle what the Voice says will be fairly easy. Your strength will be more than adequate to deal successfully with the specific triggers. When, at some future point, you have successfully dealt with level ten triggers, you will begin all over again with level one triggers. The second time around you will put the level one triggers that no longer trigger the Voice into the R.I.P. file. After working on all of the level one triggers, you will proceed to level two triggers and continue as you did before. During each cycle of moving from one to ten, you will no doubt continue to discover new triggers in your life. As you make hierarchies of them, they will be dealt with in your next go around.

Methods of Voice Provocation

Begin by taking all of the level one triggers from your Voice Box, keeping them together (using a rubber band is a simple method). You will initially be working on only one trigger at a time, so you may begin with any card in the group. (Later, when you have become adept at Voice Provocation, you can work on as many as four triggers at any one time.) Once you have chosen a specific level one trigger, your goal is to expose yourself to that trigger while fighting the Voice. You will do this until you can be master of the Voice in that trigger situation. When you have done this, put the trigger card back into the Voice Box and move on to another trigger.

By now you are aware of the fact that not all of your triggers can be so easily manipulated. The trigger "eating an extra bite at dinner" is an easy trigger to use. However, if "having someone spontaneously offer me food" is a trigger, you can see that you have very little control over this happening to you. For this reason, you need two different ways to provoke the Voice: using the real world and using your imagination.

Reality method

Before practicing Voice Provocation, you must pin down the specifics of the trigger. Where will you practice? When will you practice? Who will you practice with? If the trigger is "eating in a familiar restaurant with one close friend," then you must decide which restaurant, who the friend will be, and when you will practice the Voice Provocation. If the trigger is "looking at myself in the mirror with all my clothes on," then you must decide which mirror in which room and when you will do it. Of course, you will put this activity into your Daily Schedule.

Mental method

The reality method is always the one you want to use if it is feasible. But there will be times when it will not be possible to practice Voice Provocation on demand. For instance, if one of your triggers is "stepping on the scale and finding that I have gained 5 pounds," it will be impossible for you to do this every day. For this reason, you need to practice Voice Provocation in your imagination. Your progressive relaxation and imagery skills will be beneficial for you here. When you have relaxed your body, you can go on to imagine the trigger in vivid detail. By so doing, you will easily provoke the Voice into harassing you.

Practicing Voice Provocation

At first you should practice only one trigger a day—although you may practice it as many times in a day as you desire. When you get better at Voice Provocation, try two different triggers a day, then three, until you reach your maximum of four triggers per day. When you have gotten proficient enough to simultaneously deal with four triggers, there will still be days in which you choose to only work on one. Don't let the Voice tell you that such a choice is a step backwards or a failure.

Before working on your Voice Provocation each day, you need to complete the Daily Provocation Practice Record. On this sheet, identify which trigger or triggers you will be practicing. You should also include the variables involved in each trigger, such as where you will practice, when you will practice, who will be involved, and whether the practice will be done physically or mentally. The following record sheet should be used as part of your morning or evening ritual—you may decide to complete the record each morning or the prior evening.

Daily Provocation Practice Record

1. **WHICH** triggers will you practice?

    Voice Trigger 1 _____

    Voice Trigger 2 _____

    Voice Trigger 3 _____

    Voice Trigger 4 _____

2. **WHERE** will you practice these triggers?

    Voice Trigger 1 _____

    Voice Trigger 2 _____

    Voice Trigger 3 _____

    Voice Trigger 4 _____

3. **WHEN** will you practice these triggers?

    Voice Trigger 1 _____

    Voice Trigger 2 _____

    Voice Trigger 3 _____

    Voice Trigger 4 _____

4. **WHO** will be involved in practicing these triggers?

    Voice Trigger 1 _____

    Voice Trigger 2 _____

    Voice Trigger 3 _____

    Voice Trigger 4 _____

At the end of each day, fill out a Provocation Evaluation in order to gain as much knowledge as possible from your practice sessions.

Provocation Evaluation

1. What trick did the Voice try to use with you?

Voice Trigger 1 _____

Voice Trigger 2 _____

Voice Trigger 3 _____

Voice Trigger 4 _____

2. What did you do when it tried to trick you?

Voice Trigger 1 _____

Voice Trigger 2 _____

Voice Trigger 3 _____

Voice Trigger 4 _____

3. How did you do when it tried to confuse you?

Voice Trigger 1 _____

Voice Trigger 2 _____

Voice Trigger 3 _____

Voice Trigger 4 _____

4. How did you combat the Voice's use of speed and secrecy?

Voice Trigger 1 _____

Voice Trigger 2 _____

Voice Trigger 3 _____

Voice Trigger 4 _____

5. On a scale of one to five, how well did you do against the Voice?

Voice Trigger 1 _____

Voice Trigger 2 _____

Voice Trigger 3 _____

Voice Trigger 4 _____

Practicing Voice Provocation is a four-step process. (1) Before actually engaging in the provocation, you must fight the Voice on paper for ten minutes in an attempt to anticipate what it will say to you during your provocation. Although this may seem unnecessary with level one triggers, it is a good habit to get into before reaching the higher level triggers. (2) You must expose yourself to the trigger situation (physically or mentally) and fight the Voice during the entire provocation process. The Voice Fighting may be done either out loud or mentally, depending upon where you are at the time. The fight should take at least fifteen minutes each time. (3) When you are finished, you must spend at least five minutes telling yourself how well you did. Even if it wasn't perfect, find something good to tell yourself. This step is often the most neglected one. When you fail to congratulate yourself, the Voice will eagerly point out all the imperfections of what you just did. If you allow this to happen, you will lose the impact of Voice Provocation; you will let the Voice rob you of your triumph. (4) As mentioned previously, rate your performance on a scale of one to five. In deciding what score to give yourself, use the following guidelines:

1 - if you didn't use your Voice Fighting skills at all
2 - if you listened to the Voice more than you fought it
3 - if you listened to the Voice sometimes during Voice Fighting
4 - if you were mildly distracted by the Voice
5 - if you were in complete control of the Voice Fighting

Be careful of your self-rating. Even when you have done well, the Voice will try to trick you into giving yourself a three when you actually deserve a five. Don't feel afraid of being honest with yourself and rating yourself accordingly.

Keeping good records. Voice Provocation can often fail or succeed depending on how well you keep written records of what you have accomplished. You will be recording your self-rating in three different places. The first will be on your Daily Provocation record sheet.

You will next put the self-rating on the front of the trigger card(s) you have been using. Put the date and rating on each card—if you practiced a trigger more than once during the day, put each rating and the average on the front of the trigger card. For example, your trigger card may look like this:

Eating by myself at McDonalds		5
3/14	4, 3, 5	AVE = 4
3/15	5, 4	AVE = 4.5

Weekly Provocation Record

		1		2		3		4	
Voice Trigger									
Level	Rating								
Voice Trigger									
Level	Rating								
Voice Trigger									
Level	Rating								
Voice Trigger									
Level	Rating								
Voice Trigger									
Level	Rating								
Voice Trigger									
Level	Rating								
Voice Trigger									
Level	Rating								

Finally, you should make your self-rating part of your Weekly Provocation Record. This record is meant to give you a comparative record of your progress over a week's time. You will notice that the form has four columns, one for each trigger you are working on. When you begin you will just be using column one. At the end of each day, identify the trigger(s) you worked on, the level number, and your self-rating. This form will also help you decide when to change triggers. Your goal is to be able to earn a self-rating of four or better on a trigger for two days in a row. If you practice a trigger more than once in a given day, then use the average for your daily rating on this form. When you have attained your goal of two successive days of four or better ratings, put that trigger card back into your Voice Box and move to another trigger at the same level.

On the other hand, if you should have difficulty with the Voice on a particular trigger, it may be that the trigger should be given a higher level than you first assumed. If you cannot move above a rating of three after five consecutive days, then move that trigger into the next higher level. After you have changed the number on the trigger card, create a new trigger that is less intense to take its place.

Voice Provocation Tips

The Voice will try a number of tactics to get you to discontinue this phase. It knows that if you become routinely successful in this stage, you will win your life back and cease to be a Deadly Dieter. The following suggestions are being passed on to you by the hundreds of successful clients at my clinic who have been able to defeat the Voice in their lives.

1. **Engage in Voice Provocation with a positive attitude.** Meeting the Voice head-on is always the best long-term strategy. Even if you are not entirely successful, the opportunities for learning are enormous.

2. **Approach Voice Provocation one step at a time.** Change is always easier when done gradually. Impatience has been the downfall of more than one Deadly Dieter. Slow success is better than fast failure.

3. **Take calculated risks.** Dealing with Voice Triggers always involves some type of risk. If you are having difficulty taking a risk, read your essay on risk taking and ask yourself if you are demanding certitude in your Voice Provocation.

4. **Work on easier triggers before attempting the more difficult ones.** Success on easy triggers will strengthen you for the higher level ones. A weight lifter doesn't try to bench press his body weight until he has successfully worked on smaller weights. When he has strengthened his muscles sufficiently, graduation to heavier weights is natural. Early success builds momentum for harder triggers.

5. **Expect to succeed.** Now that you are a successful Voice fighter, defeating the Voice is no longer a wish—it is an expectation. And expectations can be self-fulfilling. Remember, also, that most of us are capable of accomplishing more than we think.

6. **Remain open to new information.** Your creativity is a powerful weapon against the Voice. The information I have given you on Voice Provocation is merely an outline. If you discover new ways of defeating the Voice, by all means use them. You may even want to write to me and share your ideas so that I can pass them on to others. This book was only possible because of people like yourself who shared their methods of success during therapy.

7. **Build and use support networks.** Any change project can be made easier if you can get others involved in the process. If your support network is weak or nonexistent, you may want to ask yourself the following questions:

   What type of support would I like to have?
   Who could provide that support?
   Where do I find this person(s)?

How do I go about getting them to support me?
Would it help to have a contract with this support person?
Do I need to practice any social skills?

Making changes when you have other people to support and encourage you is often easier than flying solo.

Voice Coping Statements

Unfortunately, life is never as neat and tidy as we would like it. No matter how well you have constructed your Voice Box and identified Voice Triggers, there will be times when you must confront a higher level trigger than the level you are currently working on. At other times, certain events may occur that surprise you by bringing on the Voice. Something may occur that you did not identify as a Voice Trigger.

When these situations occur, the Voice can immobilize you because you are not yet strong enough to defeat it in that specific situation. The Voice will get you to believe that this situation is so gigantic that a mere mortal such as you is completely incapable of dealing with it. The Voice can get you so stirred up in certain situations that your high stress level will cause you to forget everything you know about Voice Fighting. These Voice Coping Statements will help you to slow down to the point where you can pull yourself together enough to successfully fight the Voice.

Because Voice Coping Statements will help you grit your teeth and make it through any situation as best you can, they are to be used as a set of emergency tools tucked into your Voice Fighting Kit. By using them at the appropriate time, you will be able to keep your wits about you in a time-limited but strong trigger situation. However, they can work so well that it will be tempting to use them all the time instead of Voice Fighting. DON'T DO IT! They are to be used for emergency purposes only. If you find yourself using them more than several times a month, you probably need to improve the quality of your Voice Box.

Voice Coping Statements work by breaking down a "big" trigger into smaller, more manageable bits. These smaller segments are blocks of time running from the moment you are aware of the inevitability of the higher level trigger to after the trigger situation has passed. These four blocks of time are known as: preparing, confronting, coping, and relaxing. The preparing phase begins as soon as the Voice starts hassling you about the big trigger. The confronting phase starts just prior to the trigger— when it becomes imminent. The coping phase occurs while you are actually in the trigger situation. And the relaxing phase starts as soon as the trigger situation is finished. The first phase tends to be the longest, the second the shortest. But there may be times when the trigger sneaks up on you so suddenly that you have to skip phases one and two and jump directly into phase three.

To construct your emergency Voice Coping Statements, you will need four more index cards. Write the name of one of the four phases at the top of each card. You will then fill that card with sample coping statements. Read through the following samples of Voice Coping Statements for each of the four phases below. When you get an idea of what statements you would like to use, make up your own list of statements for each of the four phases. When you have completed this, put the four cards at the bottom of your Voice Fighting Kit and use them when necessary.

Voice Coping Statements

1. Preparing

There's really nothing to worry about.
Others can do it, so can I.
I've done it before, I can do it again.
Only the Voice can ruin this for me.
The issue is not the trigger, but rather the Voice.
It'll be easier once I start to fight the Voice.

2. Confronting

Stay organized—don't let the Voice muddle my thinking.
I need to slow down and take it step by step.
Any discomfort I need is a signal to fight the Voice.
Only the Voice, not the trigger, can defeat me.
It's okay not to deal with this trigger perfectly.
I can only blow it by listening to the Voice.

3. Coping

RELAX: breathe naturally, release muscle tension, calm my mind.
This trigger cannot go on forever.
I will not let tunnel vision keep me from fighting the Voice.
Losing control is merely giving in to the Voice.
Remember to keep this trigger broken down into small steps.
If I keep fighting the Voice, I will win!

4. Relaxing

I did it!
I really am stronger than the Voice.
So what if it wasn't perfect, next time will be better.
I'm going to tell about my success.
Each time I fight the Voice, I get stronger and stronger.
If I did this well now, just wait until I progress to higher levels.

Motivators

What Are Motivators?

Since the 1930s, continual research has produced a large body of factual information about human behavior. Recently, it has become apparent that there are a few laws of human behavior that can be very powerful in describing and predicting our behavior. One of these, the law of motivation, is based on a technical principle called operant conditioning. This proposition states that the consequences of our behavior can strongly motivate what we do if we control the application of these consequences in a systematic way. Once we understand the relationship between our behavior and its consequences, we can gain tremendous control over the direction our lives take.

The significance of consequences is not really a new idea. It has been around for thousands of years. The difference is that today we can now apply the influence of consequences more efficiently and effectively. There are basically two types of consequences related to our behavior: motivators (consequences that increase the frequency of our behavior) and deterrents (consequences that decrease the frequency of our behavior). We will focus only on motivators, because this use is more predictable and has longer lasting results.

There are two types of motivators: positive motivators and negative motivators. Both types can be used to increase the frequency of our behaviors. You use positive motivators when you give yourself something pleasant. Negative motivators (which are less commonly used) occur when you take something unpleasant away from yourself. With both types of motivators, you want your behavior to increase.

Categories of Motivators

Both types of motivators can be classified into three different categories: things, activities, and people. The first includes anything tangible—inanimate things that can be touched or handled, such as money, clothing, or stereos. Another category of motivators is activities—doing things that you enjoy can often be turned into a very powerful motivator. The final category of motivator is people—being around certain people or being with a special person can also be very motivating. The effectiveness of each will vary, depending on how much you want any specific motivator.

Using motivators effectively requires the following steps: (1) identifying the motivators that work for you, (2) arranging them in order of effectiveness, (3) developing a plan for using them, and (4) following the guidelines for their use.

Finding Motivators

The first step in using motivators effectively in your own life is to discover them. Many Deadly Dieters find this to be a difficult task. If your Deadly Diet has continued for any length of time, you may have forgotten how to enjoy yourself. There may be very few things in your life that you still enjoy. The Deadly Diet can also kill your enjoyment of life itself and the world around you.

To get some idea of what kind of motivators might be useful in your life, answer the following questions. Try to answer them as if you were not on the Deadly Diet. If you can still remember what life was like before going on this Diet, use this information to help you answer the questions.

If you cannot remember anything good in your past, try to answer the questions as if it were now sometime in the future and you were not a Deadly Dieter. It may even be helpful to have a close friend help you find answers to these questions.

1. What kinds of things do you like to have?

2. What are your major interests?

3. What are your hobbies?

4. Which people do you like to be with?

5. What do you like to do with these people?

6. What do you do for fun?

7. What do you do for relaxation?

8. What are some of your fantasies?

9. What makes you feel good?

10. What would be a nice present to receive?

11. What kinds of things are important to you?

12. What would you buy if you had an extra $10, $50, or $100?

13. On what do you spend your money each week?

14. What commonplace things do you do every day that are enjoyable?

15. What would you hate to lose?

To verify for yourself that you have found enough motivators to begin your motivation program, you will need to keep a record of potential motivators. Record *anything* that happens to you that you find pleasant, that you enjoy, or that makes you feel good. Note the day, the time and place, and the event associated with each motivator.

After keeping this tally for about a week, you may discover that many things you would like to have in your life as motivators are also Voice Triggers. If this is the case with you, make more hierarchies for your Voice Box. As you pass each level, you can then begin using them as motivators.

Arranging Motivators for Effectiveness

The next step is to rank-order your motivators. You may want to do this in terms of time, money, availability, or frequency. Your list can then be divided into major motivators and minor motivators. For example, a trip to Hawaii or new stereo may be a major motivator. Going to the movies or spending time with a friend would be a minor motivator.

Next, you will need to arrange these motivators into a Motivator Menu. This is done by assigning various point values to each motivator you have just identified. Look through your list of minor motivators and find the simplest ones. Assign these a value of one. Assign the rest of your minor motivators values varying from one to five. Your major motivators will be given point values between 50 and 200. These values are tentative and can be changed any time you need to update the Motivator Menu. Give yourself several days to think about your Motivator Menu so that you can feel comfortable about the values you have given each of the motivators.

Developing a Plan

Now you are ready to formulate a plan for using your motivators. The overall goal of your plan will be to use the motivators as incentives for working on your Voice Box. To initiate your plan, you award yourself credits that can then be spent on the motivators in your menu. My recommendation is that you give yourself one credit each time you practice Voice Provocation, regardless of the self-rating you give yourself. Some of my clients even give themselves an extra one-half point bonus when they have earned a self-rating of five during their provocation practice.

To establish a credit cushion, give yourself free points for two days. After that, each use of a motivator will cost you whatever point value was assigned to it. Your plan will work best if you become neither a millionaire nor a pauper. You may have to juggle the numbers during the first week or two so that you don't pile up an excessive number of credits. But you also want enough credits so that you don't have to go in the hole.

Good record keeping will again be essential for making this Motivator Plan work for you. Construct a tally sheet, similar to a checkbook register, for keeping track of points earned and points spent. Below, you will see a sample Motivator Tally Sheet.

Motivator Tally Sheet

Trigger/ Motivator	Credits Earned [+/−]	Daily Balance	Cumulative Total
Standing on scale	+1	7	12
Went to movies	-3	4	12
Ate 2100 calories today	+1	5	13
Looked in mirror twice	+2	7	15
Bought a box of chocolates	+1	8	16
Confronted my boss	+1	9 1/2	17 1/2
Stood on scale	+1	10 1/2	18 1/2
Read 50 pages in my book	-5	5 1/2	18 1/2
Looked in mirror	+1	6 1/2	19 1/2
Bought pair of jeans one size bigger	+1 1/2	8	21
Had lunch with a person at work	+1	9	22

Each time you earn credits, record them in the "credits earned" column and add them to both the "balance" column and the "cumulative total" column. When credits are spent for minor motivators, they are subtracted ONLY from the "balance" column. Major motivators are subtracted ONLY from the "cumulative total" column.

Principles for Using Motivators

An added benefit of using motivators is that when you purchase and use your motivators you have a hedge against guilt. Many Deadly Dieters feel guilty whenever they do something nice for themselves. Now you can deal with the Voice more easily because you are not getting motivators free. You have worked for them—you have earned the right to treat yourself to something pleasant.

As you continue through the coming weeks with your Motivator Plan, you will probably need to make minor adjustments to some of the plan's details. Smoothing out a plan can be a highly satisfying venture for the person who is conquering the Deadly Diet. To do so, observe the following guidelines. Like everything else you have learned up to this point, using a Motivator Plan will not be easy. It is hard work and takes a firm dedication to getting the Voice out of your life once and for all.

1. **Consistency.** Be sure to give yourself credit each time you practice Voice Provocation. If you earn your credits haphazardly, the power of your motivators will be lost.

2. **Immediacy.** Give yourself the credit as soon as you have finished with your Voice Provocation. As the time stretches out between the behavior (Voice Provocation) and the consequence (the earned credit), the motivators lose their effectiveness.

3. **Variety.** If at all possible, try to add some variety to your motivators on a weekly basis. Add new motivators, delete old ones, or make minor changes to current motivators. For example, if a particular TV program was one of your motivators, you may decide to use a different TV program after a week or two. Or if an enjoyable activity was being used, you might want to make the activity last longer, do it in a different place, or with a different person. Variety will keep your motivators from getting stale and losing their power.

4. **Effectiveness.** If you are not receiving much pleasure from some of your motivators, feel free to get rid of them. There is nothing magic in choosing a specific motivator. Technically, motivators are only motivators if they work. So, if a motivator is not working for you, there is no need to waste your time with it.

5. **Clarity.** Make sure the terms of your motivator are clear to you. If the method of use or manner of usage is vague, you will not get maximum benefit from the motivator. Use the four criteria for goal setting in chapter three as guidelines. Is the motivator specific? Is it positively stated? Is it measurable? Is it reasonable?

6. **Frequency.** Be sure to spend your credits on your motivators as often as you can. Daily spending is a good plan. You might want to think of dividing your minor motivators into those that you can spend daily, weekly, and monthly.

7. **Honesty.** Use motivators only when you have the credits to spend. If a movie is one of your minor motivators, then you will dilute your plan by going to the movies even when you don't have the credits for doing so.

Skills Checklist

☐ Identify Voice Triggers

☐ Create hierarchies

☐ Construct Voice Box

☐ Begin Voice Provocation at level one

☐ Keep good records
   a. Daily Provocation Practice Record
   b. Provocation Evaluation

☐ Use Voice Coping Statements as a last resort

☐ Discover your personal motivators

☐ Use motivators to increase your Voice Provocation

10

Maintenance Issues

I must not fear.
Fear is the mind-killer.
Fear is the little-death that brings total obliteration.
I will face my fear.
I will permit it to pass over me and through me.
And when it is gone past
I will turn the inner eye to see its path.
Where the fear has gone there will be nothing.
Only I will remain.

—FRANK HERBERT, *DUNE*, 1965

Progress is only successful if it can be maintained for an extended period of time. As humans, we value accomplishments that are sustained, rather than those that come and go. The athlete who makes his mark early in his career but does nothing significant after that is one who is soon forgotten. It is the athlete who consistently keeps up a certain level of behavior who is remembered.

Many good behavior-change programs in the mental health field fall down in this area of follow-up and maintenance. You may know of people who have learned to quit smoking or lose weight, only to fall back into the old habits within a short period of time.

Much psychological research says that success in new behaviors must continue for at least a year in order for them to be considered adequately learned. Once the new behaviors and skills have been learned, the next six to twelve months are similar to a recovery period after a major illness. You are susceptible, at this time, to setbacks and backsliding.

Some people who have gone through our program have tricked themselves into believing that little or no work was necessary when they had finished the program. Nothing could be further from the truth. If you put in less work after you have finished this book than you did while learning its skills, then you are setting yourself up for the plateau effect.

The plateau effect can occur during this critical period because you have experienced some success against the Voice and are now beginning to enjoy the fruits of your labor. You have even begun to forget what it was that made you successful. Almost all people who find themselves on this plateau eventually find that the plateau slopes backward. This rude awakening will come when you have a setback.

Setbacks are fairly common, so you need not be surprised when you have one. They often happen soon after a series of "good days." When you have a setback, it will come as a shock because you have forgotten how powerful the Voice can be. To either forestall or lessen the impact of setbacks, you need to be aware of the Voice even when things are going well for you. When you are enjoying life, it is easy to kick back and enjoy your new-found freedom. Yet, the Voice always tries to sneak back. It is of the utmost importance you follow my often repeated guideline: ON GOOD DAYS, YOU WORK TWICE AS HARD.

You need to be on the watch for several more years—if not the rest of your life. If you can be aware of the danger signals, then it will be easier for you to prevent the Voice from bringing on a major setback in your life.

Danger Signals

There are six basic danger signals that you will constantly need to watch for: social isolation, physiological change, environmental change, lack of structure, addiction withdrawal, and personal unawareness.

Social Isolation

As we have already seen, the Voice can play havoc with the social life of a Deadly Dieter. Withdrawing from friends or not reaching out to make new friends are common problems for the Deadly Dieter. This habit can return when you are undergoing something stressful or trying to cope with some difficult situation. It is ironic that these are the very times when you need to have other people support and encourage you—yet this is when the Voice will try to convince you to isolate yourself.

Failure to reach out for help is often the result of two very common excuses: "I'm too embarrassed to admit that I have slipped" and "This issue is too trivial to bother someone about." The first excuse assumes that others expect you to be perfect. The second tries to pretend that you only need help from your friends after the roof has fallen in. Your friends will appreciate you for your honesty if you can openly admit your imperfections. Also, it is much better to reach out too soon than too late.

Physiological Change

The Voice often has a field day when things happen inside your body. Fatigue and illness are very common starting points for setbacks. When your body is tired, it is much easier for the Voice to harass you because it knows that you may be too tired to fight back.

Illness is even worse because life often comes to a grinding halt. You don't work, clean house, go to the movies, eat properly, talk with friends, or do any of the other routine things in your day. Being ill throws you off schedule. Your goals and attempts at managing your time goes askew. Sometimes when you have built up a good positive inertia, illness can put you back to ground zero.

Environmental Change

Anything that happens to you to upset your normal, everyday routine can act as an inroad for the Voice. Major events such as job changes, relationship changes, financial changes, or health changes are especially critical. And the change doesn't have to be a negative one. Were you to win the Irish Sweepstakes, the Voice would have a marvelous opportunity for pulling you down. Some of my clients have done well until they returned from a wonderful vacation. As soon as they got back, they had a setback. I'm not saying that all changes will automatically trigger a setback. You just need to be careful and watchful during these times.

Lack of Structure

You know that unstructured times have generally been difficult for you in the past. It is no different now. When my clients have setbacks, the first things they stop doing are the daily schedule and the daily rituals. Lack of structure makes your days melt into one another. It can string together so many bad days that you lose complete control over your time and your life. Remember, of course, that I am referring to a lack of internal structure, not external structure. The best structure is one that you impose from the inside, not one that has been imposed upon you from the outside.

Addiction Withdrawal

Becoming an ex-Deadly Dieter is similar to becoming an ex-addict. The Voice has had such a stranglehold on your life that you will never be like you were before the Deadly Diet. You must always remind yourself of what it was like to be a complete slave to the Voice. Withdrawal from any abusive substance is extremely painful and torturously slow. Often the addict finds it easier to go back into the addiction than to continue fighting it. Most addiction experts agree that it takes at least a year of being clean from a drug before the body has completely readapted itself. Your maintenance program is a program of addiction withdrawal and nothing less.

Fighting the addiction takes as much work and training as any other difficult task, whether it be an athletic contest or a music recital. You will have to put considerable time and effort into planning and practice.

Personal Unawareness

Perhaps all the other danger signals can be summed up in this one. By forgetting to continually monitor your environment and yourself, you are vulnerable to tunnel vision. Tunnel vision is related to Voice-avoiding busyness. Ignoring the Voice ANYTIME is dangerous. To do so means you cannot concentrate on what it is saying to you. Tunnel vision occurs anytime you are just concentrating on (1) what is happening to you, (2) what you are feeling, and (3) what you are doing. Although these things can be important, they can divert your attention away from the Voice.

Even when you are tuning in to your emotions, you need to accurately label the emotions that you are experiencing. Not knowing a constructive from a destructive emotion is a sure road to emotional confusion. Emotional confusion can upset your thinking to the point that you don't even hear the lies from the Voice. If you don't realize that your discomfort comes from a destructive emotion, you may find yourself slipping back into "discomfort dodging."

Being unaware of a potentially hazardous situation can quickly throw you into a tailspin. Adequate preparation is necessary, since anything new can leave you unprepared for the triggering effect it may have on your life. Anticipation can be a powerful tool when used for new situations.

Infrequent Voice Triggers may leave you unaware of their existence until it is too late. For many Deadly Dieters, resentment is a destructive emotion less common than any of the other five. Resentment is often forgotten just because it is so rare. Surprisingly, however, this one can pop up unexpectedly even after you have made significant progress with your life.

Setbacks

A setback happens when the Voice takes advantage of you in a way you thought would no longer happen. For example, if you have not been depressed for over a month and are hit with a big depression, that is a setback. Setbacks are always unexpected. They are also inevitable. That is why it is so important for you to learn how to handle them.

Dealing with Deadly Diet setbacks is akin to dealing with any other kind of setback. A baseball player who is in a batting slump goes back to the basics. He works on holding the bat comfortably, standing correctly, swinging the bat properly. This is all done very slowly so as to correct any bad habits that have snuck in.

Characteristics of Setbacks

Unrealistic expectations. Setbacks can immediately trigger all sorts of unrealistic expectations. The most dangerous one is that of looking for a magic solution. One of the first things people think of during a setback is "This approach isn't working anymore. I have to find something else that works better." The fallacy here is that the approach *is* working, because you have made it this far.

Extreme thinking. It is also possible that, after a period of success, you may slip back into extreme thinking. You stop letting yourself make mistakes. You begin to creep toward the belief that your goal in life is to be perfect. Of course, this is impossible, even for you! Perfectionism only allows you to be an absolute success or an absolute failure. You need to dare to be average. Average doesn't mean mediocre or bland but rather somewhere—anywhere—between the extremes.

The Great Abyss. This is often the last great step for many Deadly Dieters. When the Voice has almost been defeated, it will remind you that the new you is unfamiliar, but the old you is at least a known quantity. It will try to get you to believe that when you finally decide to completely overthrow the Deadly Diet, you will be falling into a great unknown abyss, a vast chasm that is terrifying and dangerous. The Deadly Diet has been like all the things we are familiar with—safe, comfortable, predictable, and secure. Your new life will not have any of these qualities, says the Voice. The Voice will try to convince you that to give up the Deadly Diet is to die an emotional death, to make yourself vulnerable to something larger than yourself.

Again, as is always the case with the Voice, it is telling you only part of the truth. As you look ahead, it tells you there is nothing but blackness and emptiness without the Deadly Diet. The truth is that there is no abyss, no void for you to fall into. When you penetrate the blackness ahead of you, you will see green grass, blue sky, and a beautiful life.

Developing an Emergency Plan

By far the most effective strategy for setbacks is one of prevention. When things are going well for you, concentrate on those skills that will maintain your momentum. Some of these skills are described for you in the next section, "Positive Progress." But no matter how well you try to avoid setbacks, they are inevitable. You need to have another line of defense for when they come.

You can prepare an Emergency Plan by providing yourself with visual cues, both stationary and portable. The stationary cues can be put on large poster board or some other large surface. Place your poster where you can easily see it in your house, apartment, or room. You also need to put your Emergency Plan on an index card to carry it with you at all times. It may be wise to put it in the bottom of your Voice Fighting Kit, maybe even in another color so that you can find it quickly if needed.

On the front of the card, put the following questions:

- What game is the Voice playing?
- What triggered the Voice?
- Do I want to change what is happening to me?
- When do I want to change?
- What tools shall I use to make the change?
- How can I motivate myself to make this change?

On the back of the card (or the bottom of the poster board), put a list of your available tools for pulling you out of the setback:

- Breathe naturally
- Release my muscle tension
- Calm my mind
- Identify destructive emotions
- Identify Voice Key Words
- Fight the Voice on paper
- Use affirmations after defeating the Voice
- Put this trigger in my Voice Box

Positive Progress

Life is more than constantly being on your guard for setbacks and fighting them when they come. I want you to spend a major portion of your time moving forward and enjoying the continuing progress of personal growth. The skills necessary to keep your progress on a positive note include (1) goal setting, (2) personal control, and (3) increasing personal awareness.

Goal Setting

Goal setting is the basis for an active and enjoyable life. The mightiest ship in the world will destroy itself if it has no direction. This does not mean that your life must be rigid and inflexible. Goal setting merely provides the framework upon which to hang your spontaneity and creativity.

In a maintenance program there are many things you can use to enhance goal setting: a daily schedule, a daily checklist, a weekly checklist, a monthly checklist, anticipatory plans, healing time, and an activity list.

Daily schedule. Whenever you feel overwhelmed or helpless, chances are you have slacked off on using your daily schedule. One of the first things I check when someone calls me about a small backward step is how they are using their daily schedule. Ten times out of ten, they have been negligent in its use. Your daily schedule will help you to pull out of confusion and to keep your progress positive. It does this by helping you to minimize surprises, procrastination, and the setting of unreasonable goals.

As part of your maintenance program, you need to be "creatively busy" as opposed to "distractingly busy." In the past, you tended to busy yourself in order to distract yourself from the Voice. You now know that this is basically useless. However, this does not mean that being busy is, by itself, a bad thing. Filling your life with activities and people that help you to explore your potential is a lot different than madly keeping your mind busy to escape the Voice. You might want to consider sports, self-help groups, volunteer work, a new vocation, hobbies, crafts, or special interest groups. But remember: take one day at a time.

Daily checklist. One of your evening rituals, the Success Journal, can now be converted to a daily checklist. At the end of each day, identify those skills that you were able to practice during that day. An example of one such checklist follows.

Daily Checklist

Date_____

☐ Morning rituals   ☐ Taking risks

☐ Evening rituals   ☐ Correctly identifying my emotions

☐ Voice Fighting   ☐ Breathing

☐ Identifying Voice Key Words   ☐ Muscle relaxation

☐ Mind calming   ☐ Using affirmations

☐ Exercising my rights

☐ Taking personal respon-
sibility

☐ Using realistic expectations

☐ Getting my needs met

☐ Voice Provocation

☐ Using Motivators

☐ Reviewing material in this book

Weekly checklist. Concentrating on your daily accomplishments alone can keep your vision too narrow. It really is hard to see the forest for the trees. For this reason, looking at your life in weekly segments will help you to find a perspective in your daily affairs. Most people have found it helpful to have a regular time to do this You may want to mark your calendar at the end or the beginning of your week. For example, Sunday afternoon or evening would be a good time to check your weekly progress. The purpose of this activity is to help you smooth out the small ups and downs of daily existence. By looking at your life over the course of a week, you can ignore some of the minor setbacks yet still see your general direction and take any necessary corrective action before it is too late.

You'll need about thirty minutes to complete your Weekly Checklist. You may want to make it look something like this:

Weekly Checklist

Date_____

My success for this past week:
>   a.
>   b.
>   c.

Which key words has the Voice played with me this week?
>   a.
>   b.
>   c.

This past week I have learned:

I will review the following pages in this book next week:_____

I will do the following things for myself this week in order to help myself grow:
>   a.
>   b.
>   c.

I will work on the following Voice Triggers this week:

Monthly checklist. You can gain a still wider perspective on yourself by taking stock of broader personal areas on a monthly basis. Do this by asking yourself the following questions in a monthly checklist:

1. What progress have I made against the Voice?
2. What progress have I made emotionally?
3. What progress have I made intellectually?
4. What progress have I made spiritually?
5. What progress have I made physically?

Anticipatory planning. If you have been invited to a party that almost guarantees enormous amounts of food, you will find the situation—and the Voice—much easier to deal with if you have made plans before attending the party. Your plan needs to revolve around these five steps: (l) gathering information, (2) exploring your options, (3) developing a specific plan, (4) using your plan, and (5) evaluating your plan.

For the upcoming party, you would want to know how many people will be there, what kind of and how much food will be served, how many people you will know, what the physical layout of the location is, how long it will last, and who you will be going with.

Your options will depend upon this information. Basically, your options include talking or not talking to certain people, eating the foods you are comfortable with, taking time to reduce stress and fight the Voice, and deciding when to arrive and when to leave.

For each of these options, you can plan in advance what you want to do. You may even want to have a back-up plan in case the first one becomes impractical. If you have any questions on how you can get what you want, ask your support person or group, therapist, or friend.

To actually carry off your plan, allow time to regroup or slow yourself down should it be necessary. Bathrooms, patios, and even coatrooms are good places to grab a few private minutes for yourself. Bring notes on index cards to help remind you of your strategy.

After the party, spend time reviewing the entire event. What did you do right? How did the Voice get you or try to get you? How were you effective against it? What new things did you learn? How can you reward yourself for doing a good job? How can you do better next time in a similar situation?

Healing time. Finally, goal setting is related to patience. Some goals are not meant to be completed quickly. The Voice has had a stranglehold on your life for a long time. You need to give yourself the benefit of healing time. Most people need at least one to three years to remove most of the major emotional scars that the Voice has inflicted. Recovering from the Deadly Diet is similar to recovering from a major illness or to the withdrawal an addict experiences when drying out. And we all know that old habits die hard—if at all. I suspect that the Voice will never leave. It is built into our human nature. As you grow and regain control of your life, let your feelings become a part of your life without ever again trusting them. To make decisions based on your feelings is to open the door wide and invite the Voice back into your life.

Activity list. Assume that there will be times in your life when you will become bored. In the past, the Voice has used this feeling to take advantage of you. To prevent this and to deal constructively with "nothing to do," you will want to build an activity list. Include things that you enjoy on a regular basis, things you enjoy but never have enough time for, and things that you might enjoy but never have been able to try. The following is a sample activity list.

Activity List

Always	*Rarely*	*Never*
Jigsaw puzzles	Read a "trashy" novel	Take a train ride
Lying in the sun	Watch the soaps	Test-drive a new car
Talking to friends on the phone	Take an adult ed class	Ask a male friend out on a date
Shopping	Just sit and think	Go skiing
Drive in the country	Sew a new outfit	Go camping
Macrame		Attend an opera
Needlepoint		

Control

Control is the key issue in your fight against the Voice and the ravages of the Deadly Diet. Remember that control does not mean being "uptight, rigid, and inflexible," but rather the ability to determine your own destiny and make your own choices.

Control of your inner life. In America, we tend to trivialize our language by looking at words as a mere means to an end. We use words carelessly, repetitiously, and incorrectly. Writers of fantasy-type fiction, such as Tolkien and LeGuin, treat words and their use as very special. To them, words have a power rooted in deep mystery. People in their stories who are careless in their choice of words often find themselves in situations nightmarishly difficult. Words have the power to enslave others or unlock long forgotten mysteries.

Although our scientific framework of the universe doesn't allow us to accept these fantasies as part of our working reality, we must still acknowledge the power of words. They are symbols that often carry greater weight than the immediate context. For example, "fat" is a simple word that any English-speaker can easily understand. It is also an ambiguous word whose meaning depends upon what the standard of measure happens to be at the moment. Any person, no matter how small, is "fat" compared to a broomstick. On the other hand, we are all "skinny" compared to an elephant.

These obvious characteristics of the word "fat" are lost on the Deadly Dieter, who transforms its relative meaning to an absolute one. At first, having *any* fat on one's body becomes unthinkable. Later, the mere thought of "being fat" can send the Deadly Dieter into a frenzy.

Many Deadly Dieters are deeply afraid that when they give up the Deadly Diet they will automatically become "fat." This anxiety may be what keeps you from wholeheartedly involving yourself in getting rid of the problem. This type of thinking is another example of extremist, black-and-white thinking. The world is not divided into thin people and fat people. The opposite of thin is not fat. Thin and fat are similar in the sense that both are an extreme position. The opposite of both of them is a word called "normal." "Thin" must be seen as being in the same category as "fat." As extreme words, "thin" and "fat" can be unforgiving tyrants keeping you from seeing the world and yourself in more realistic terms.

Other words that commonly provide obstacles for the Deadly Dieter are "normal," "lonliness," "discomfort," "binge," "good," "bad," and "mistake." If you find that certain words are powerful Voice Triggers in your life, you will want to defuse them.

Defusing these words means learning their true meaning. This is done by using standards generally accepted by society at large. If the Voice has dominated your life for a long time, you may have forgotten what these standards are. One of your standard references can be a good dictionary. For example, you may define "thin" as "happy." The dictionary will tell you that thinness has nothing to do with happiness. In fact, a thesaurus lists the following words as similar to "thin:"

slim	gaunt
poor	scrawny
sparse	feeble
rarified	

If you study these words carefully, you will notice that none of them are particularly attractive words. Each time your Voice tries to talk about being "thin," you can get a better perspective on your life by using one of these other words instead. None of my clients enjoy being called "scrawny" or "gaunt."

Visual input is also helpful in learning the meaning of words. If you still look at your skinny self in the mirror and see yourself as "fat" or "normal," then you might want to compare yourself to what society sees as fat or normal. You can get a very good idea of what society considers a good-looking woman by looking through the pictures in a men's magazine—for example, *Playboy*. The women displayed on those pages are not there because they are gaunt or scrawny.

One of my extremely thin clients used pictures from magazines to help her redefine her concept of reality. She did this by drawing a line along the bottom of a poster board and marking on it a scale running from one to ten. Looking through several magazines, she found pictures of extremely skinny women. Over number one on the scale she put some pictures of these scrawny—and not very attractive—women. On the right side of the scale, she placed pictures of very obviously obese women. Above five she set pictures of women from *Playboy* who tended to match her coloring and bone structure.

Then, as she stood naked in front of her mirror, she compared her body with those in the pictures. She was shocked that she could only rate herself a two on the skinny-fat scale. She is now beginning to realize that she can choose to have the body weight of the women in the middle, rather than those on either end.

You need to redefine *all* the words and standards used by the Voice. This can be done for clothing size, calorie intake, and amount of exercise. Don't let the Voice tell you that a certain clothing size is related to your worthfulness or that caloric intake must be rigidly controlled.

Sometimes the Voice may even accurately point out something about yourself that is less than perfect. Whenever the Voice gleefully points out a real liability in your life, you can say to it, "Thanks, Voice, I'll work on that one!"

Control of your outer life. You can control not only your concepts, ideas, and images, but also those things that other people can see and hear. That is, you can control your communication, your emotions, and your behavior. If you want to improve your communication skills, I recommend that you read and study the book *Messages*, by McKay, Davis, and Fanning. Your emotions can be controlled by correctly labelling them as constructive or destructive as they occur. You can control your behavior by learning new social skills and continuing your work with the Voice Box. Even some seemingly impossible situations are within your control. They are within your control because you ALWAYS have choices. For instance, in any uncomfortable situation you can always (1) stay and be uncomfortable, (2) stay and be comfortable, (3) leave and be comfortable, and (4) leave and be uncomfortable.

You can learn to control the behaviors of eating and weighing properly. There are countless books on good eating habits. Nutritionists are trained to help you learn these skills. Using these resources only strengthens your hand—it doesn't weaken it, as the Voice would have you believe. For many, the scale looms as a vicious monster ready to devour any sense of self-confidence gained in previous days. This is silly! The scale is only a mechanical device. You are its master and need not be intimidated by its presence or what reading it gives you.

In developing more control over your life, you will find that two weapons will begin to emerge as powerful allies against the Voice: humor and boredom. That's right. Boredom can be very advantageous if used properly. You know that the Voice is repetitious. Sometime in the future, the Voice will try to hit you with some bit of nonsense, and you will find yourself yawning and saying to yourself, "Oh, no. Not this twaddle again." When this happens, enjoy it. It means that you have begun to internalize Voice Fighting so that it is barely even conscious anymore. The same holds true for laughter. You may find yourself chuckling or giggling over what the Voice has just said to you. Don't be afraid of your laughter. If used naturally, it is a deadly defense against the Voice's attempted intrusion.

Steps To Increase Personal Awareness

Awareness of what is happening to you both internally and externally is a skill you have been developing since the beginning of this book. Continue to be aware of your Voice Triggers. Watch for such things as loneliness, boredom, fatigue, insecurity, doubt, stress, taking risks, and deprivation.

Consequences are very powerful, and you can use them to your advantage. Continue to remind yourself of the consequences of being a Deadly Dieter. Then compare these consequences with those of being an ex-Deadly Dieter. Would you rather have the consequences of isolation, separation, failure, and being out of control? Or do joy, self-esteem, growth, and peace appeal to you?

Many Deadly Dieters eventually need to come to grips with their own sexuality. Since the Deadly Diet usually has its roots in the teen years, it is not surprising that sexual distortions are also present. What teenager has not wrestled with his or her own emerging and powerful sexual needs? These new sensations can be put aside and camouflaged by the Deadly Diet. Awareness of and honesty about your true sexual needs can help you to round out your entire personality.

The following guidelines have been garnered from my clients over the years. They are suggestions that others have used to help in maintaining personal progress. You may find it helpful to read them over on a weekly basis.

1. Be willing to change. "The only thing permanent in life is change." This idea is thousands of years old, yet still has meaning for you today. Ask yourself, "Am I living in a way that is deeply satisfying to me and which truly expresses me?" By accepting change as exciting instead of scary, you automatically open new doors for yourself daily.

2. Take responsibility. Be willing to accept the consequences of your behavior without blame or excuse. Refuse to indulge in self-pity when life hands you a raw deal. Accept the fact that nobody gets through life without some sorrow and misfortune.

3. Be willing to take risks. The biggest risk of all is to take no risks. Begin to see risks as your opportunity for growth. Growth and change can only be accomplished by testing your limits; this means taking risks. And taking risks is scary. However, it is okay to be scared as long as you continue to take the risk.

4. Experience life honestly and directly. This means not living in the past nor too far into the future. It is easy to dwell on what might have been or what could be. Wishful thinking is one of the most common barriers to personal growth. You need to trust yourself enough to accept all kinds of information about yourself without having to distort it. Honesty means seeing yourself as others see you. It means the willingness to admit you are wrong, that you make mistakes, that you act irresponsibly. Try to see things as they are, not as you would like them to be.

5. Allow yourself more positive experiences. The good things in life don't just happen. You can bring them about by knowing what you want and then getting it. As you increase your movement toward positive things and decrease your movement away from negative things, life begins to take on a new freshness and excitement.

6. Be prepared to be different. Cultivate the old-fashioned virtues: love, honor, compassion, and loyalty. This may mean that you will be different from what others in your life want you to be. Be prepared to be unpopular when your views don't agree with theirs. Trust your own thoughts and accept your uniqueness. Stop being what others want you to be and start being who you want to be.

7. Get involved. Find something bigger than yourself to believe in. Life is more than the island we live on. It often seems that most people are interested only in themselves and their immediate surroundings. Force yourself to stay involved with the real world. Resist the temptation to withdraw and let the Voice run your life during periods of stress and confusion.

8. Slow down. Self-improvement takes time. A certain portion of your time needs to be spent in contemplation and self-exploration. When you spin your wheels, you make more mistakes and let the Voice back into your life. You will get more done with your life going at a slower pace than you will if you zip through life at breakneck speed.

9. Monitor your life. Information is vital to your growth. The written records you used during this book helped you sort out the confusion in your personal growth. By writing down your goals, you made them clearer and thus easier to reach. But don't expect *too* much of yourself. You want to avoid too wide a gap between your expectations and your ability to meet your goals. Better to meet a smaller goal than not meet a bigger one.

10. Assess your progress regularly. Progress is another relative word—it has no meaning unless compared to something else. No one ever finally "arrives." Progress is a process which continues until your death. Nor is it measured by looking to see how much further you have to go; it is measured by looking back to see how far you have come.

Maturity

Maturity is the process in which you make full use of your talents, capacities, and human potentialities. It is something that is impossible to even consider as long as the Voice is running your life. However, now that you have regained control of your life, you need to begin looking forward rather than back. Striving after maturity means that you will be forced to emphasize the brighter side of human nature. You will begin to reach beyond yourself toward that receding horizon that gets farther away from you the closer you get. Maturity is a goal that no human being ever reaches because the goals are far beyond our finite capabilities. Yet, the striving for the goal of maturity is an endeavor worthy of all human beings.

It is a lifestyle that is the exact opposite of the one run by the Voice. As a person reaching for maturity, you become more aware of your assets and positive qualities. By being more aware of who you really are, you become more capable of getting your personal needs met. As maturity becomes a part of your new life, you become more willing to accept yourself for who you really are. This allows you to more easily expand your range of experiences in the real world—as opposed to living in the fantasy world created by the Voice. As you grow, your autonomy and self-sufficiency increases. Your own human creativity is something that becomes more and more accessible to you.

Characteristics of Maturity

If you are interested in pursuing the goal of maturity, it is important to more clearly identify the components that make up this goal. Although

I have identified nine such parts, you may also notice other aspects that I have missed.

Perceptual efficiency. Maturity allows you to luckily sort out your emotions and identify the destructive ones that are polluting your constructive emotions. As a mature person, you know your rights, accept responsibility, have realistic expectations, know your needs, and take reasonable risks.

Acceptance of reality. You can accept yourself, others, and human nature with all its flaws and shortcomings as they are. This is not the same as being fatalistic. Rather you accept these things as obstacles to be worked around. Just as you accept the fact that water is wet and rocks are hard, you accept the fact that people (including yourself) are inconsistent, forgetful, and fallible.

Naturalness. As a mature person you spend little time trying to create an effect for people. You can be yourself even when it makes others uncomfortable. Yet, you do not deliberately try to annoy others. You are able to enter into the little ceremonies and rituals of life with good humor and a gracefulness that may reveal your personal opinions.

Detachment and privacy. Because of your maturity, you can enjoy solitude and time alone. By learning to take control from the Voice, you have also learned to rely on your own personal judgment. You can enjoy your own company and do not need the constant stimulation of others to make you happy. When you do spend time with people, your relationship is based on choice rather than dependency, loneliness, insecurity, or manipulation .

Constructive motivation. The more mature you become, the more you rely on internal instead of external motivators. Rather than relying on other people's beliefs and cultural pressures, much of your motivation comes from within.

Freshness of appreciation. Your "rebirth" gives you a new capacity to appreciate the basic goodness of life. This is something that can happen over and over again. This appreciation may be experienced as awe, pleasure, wonder, and even possibly ecstasy.

Empathy. Since true maturity only comes after one has struggled with pain and suffering, you are able to more readily identify with the distress and afflictions of those around you. As a result, your conflicts with others tend to be more problem-oriented now than people-oriented as they were in the past. You can "disagree without being disagreeable." Empathy also allows you to accept the differences between yourself and other people.

Natural intimacy. Because you can be honest with yourself, your friendships are also characterized by openness and honesty. Intimacy is also fostered by the fact that you have friends because you *want* them— not because you *need* them.

Personal ethical standards. By questioning the Voice's "shoulds," you have also questioned the standards passed on to you by others. The standards that remain are *your* standards, the result of much careful thinking and reasoning. But even though your standards are strong and definite, you do not assume that they are either absolute or better than those of others.

Remember that these characteristics are not meant to push you back into a perfectionistic mold. These are ideals that none of us will ever entirely reach. Yet, the striving for them is what life is all about. These characteristics are also not meant to paint a black-and-white picture of life. Mature people still have silly, wasteful, or thoughtless habits. Mature people can be boring, stubborn, irritating, and subject to temper tantrums. In all honesty, we must admit that the mature person will never be totally altruistic or totally free from personal pride or vanity. Mature people will continue to be partial to their own activities, ideas, family, and friends.

Resources

Be resourceful. When you need help, find out where to go—and go there. We have compiled at The California Clinic a moderate listing of books and services. If you know of a resource missed in the listing, please contact us and we will add it to our listing.

Services

American Anorexia/Bulimia Association, Inc.
133 Cedar Lane
Teaneck, NJ 07666

Anorexia Nervosa Aid Society (ANAS)
Box 213
Lincoln Center, Mass. 01733

Anorexia Nervosa and Related Eating Disorders (ANRED)
P.O. Box 5102
Eugene, Oregon 97405

Associates for Bulimia and Related Disorders
31 West 10th Street
New York, NY 10011

Bulimia Anorexia Self-Help, Inc. (BASH)
522 North New Ballas Road, Suite 206
Saint Louis, MO 63141

Center for the Study of Anorexia
    1 West 91st Street
    New York, NY 10024

Columbia Presbyterian Medical Center
    Eating Disorders Research and Treatment Program
    NY State Psychiatric Institute
    722 West 168th Street
    New York, NY 10032

Consuming Passions (Newsletter)
    Fulfillment Etc., Inc.
    P. O. Box 77
    Norwood, NJ 07648

Dieters Counseling Service, Inc.
    425 E. 51st Street, Suite 6E
    New York, NY 10022

Eating Disorder Program
    New York Hospital—Cornel Center
    University Medical Center
    Westchester—21 Bloomingdale Road
    White Plains, NY 10605

Eating Disorder Projects
    Michael Reese Medical Center
    Psychosomatic and Psychiatric Institute
    29th Street and Ellis Avenue
    Chicago, IL 60616

Eating Disorders Clinic
    Department of Psychiatry, M.L. #559
    University of Cincinnati
    Cincinnati, OH 45267

Eating Disorders Program
    Boulder Memorial Hospital
    311 Mapleton Avenue
    Boulder, CO 80302

Eating Disorders Unit
    Eden Hospital
    20103 Lake Chabot Road
    Castro Valley, CA 94546

John Hopkins Hospital Eating and Weight Disorder Clinic
    Meyer 3-181
    600 N. Wolfe Street
    Baltimore, MD 20200

Maryland Association for Anorexia Nervosa and Bulimia, Inc. (MAANA)
222 Gateswood Road
Lutherville, MD 21093

National Anorexia Aid Society (NAAS)
P.O. Box 29461
Columbus, OH 43229

National Association of Anorexia and Associated Disorders
Box 271
Highland Park, IL 60035

San Luis Obispo Eating Disorder Program
1652 Hansen Lane
San Luis Obispo, CA 93401

Southpark Psychology
Joseph S. Maciejko, Ph.D.
2100-52nd Avenue
Moline, IL 61265

The California Clinic
4095 Bridge St.
Fair Oaks, CA 95628

The Eating Disorders Institute
Methodist Hospital
P.O. Box 650
Minneapolis, MN 55440

The Renfrew Center
475 Spring Lane
Philadelphia, PA 19128

University of California, Los Angeles
Eating Disorder Program
Neuropsychiatric Institute
760 Westwood Plaza
Los Angeles, CA 90024

University of Minnesota Hospital
Behavioral Health Clinic
Box 393, Mayo Memorial Building
420 Delaware Street, S.E.
Minneapolis, MN 55455

Finding a Therapist

If none of the services listed for the Deadly Diet are in your area, you
need to do some digging. Now that the problem has received so much

attention, many unqualified therapists are jumping on the bandwagon and saying that they work with the problem. Many of them just apply the same techniques they have been using for other problems. To help weed out unqualified therapists, the following steps may help:

1. Write to any of the organizations listed—many of them keep referral lists. Even so, be cautious of even these referrals. Almost none of them are screened in any form. Even when they are, these screening procedures are often inefficient.

2. Call a local college or university and talk to a cognitive-behavioral psychologist. This person may help steer you away from the old-fashioned therapy approaches that do not work well with eating disorders.

3. Talk to a school nurse. These people see this problem all the time and can tell if a resource is available. If it is, they may even give you their opinion of how well it helps.

4. The Yellow Pages and local psychological referral services are not of much help. Any psychologist can put anything into a Yellow Page advertisement. Referral services are loose-knit economic organizations meant to generate income for the psychologists running them.

5. When you think you have found a therapist, ask the following questions:

   a. How long have you been treating this problem?

   b. How many people have you worked with?

   c. Can I talk with some of your former clients? (A good therapist will be more than willing to help you do this.)

   d. How long does therapy generally last? (The major bulk of therapy should last four to six months with a hard-working client.)

   e. What is your degree and where did you get it?

   f. What does your therapy consist of?
   (What does the therapist do?)

   g. What do people actually do in therapy?
   (What does the client do?)

   h. What kind of follow-up do you use after therapy is finished?
   (What are the maintenance procedures?)

   i. What are the general goals of therapy?
   (Are they specific or just vague mumbo-jumbo?)

j. How often must a person come in for therapy? (Although once per week is traditional, the decision depends on the client's time, finances, etc.)

When you think you have found a therapist, go for the first visit as if you were going on an exploration. Visiting a therapist once doesn't obligate you. After all, if the therapist can't handle your not coming back, you wouldn't want such an easily offended person for a therapist anyway. To help you evaluate the therapist's competency, complete the following questionnaire after the first visit.

How To Choose a Therapist

As a consumer of psychological services it is important that you be able to intelligently decide who you want to help you solve your problems. Dr. Arnold Lazarus is a psychologist who devised a questionnaire to help people make this decision. The following questions can help you find a therapist to make the changes in your life that you want. Use the five-point scale below in rating each of the following statements.

4 - This statement is true.
3 - It is true most of the time.
2 - It is true some of the time.
1 - It is seldom true.
0 - It is never true.

_____ 1. I feel comfortable with the therapist.

_____ 2. The therapist seems comfortable with me.

_____ 3. The therapist is casual and informal rather than stiff and formal.

_____ 4. The therapist does not treat me as if I am sick, defective, and about to fall apart.

_____ 5. The therapist is flexible and open to new ideas rather than pursuing one point of view.

_____ 6. The therapist has a good sense of humor and a pleasant disposition.

_____ 7. The therapist is willing to tell me how he/she feels about me.

_____ 8. The therapist admits limitations and does not pretend to know things he/she doesn't know.

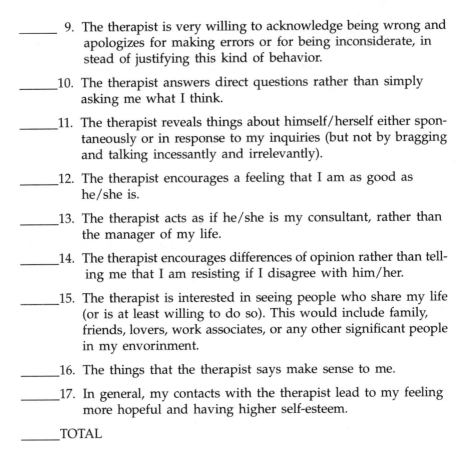

_____ 9. The therapist is very willing to acknowledge being wrong and apologizes for making errors or for being inconsiderate, in stead of justifying this kind of behavior.

_____10. The therapist answers direct questions rather than simply asking me what I think.

_____11. The therapist reveals things about himself/herself either spontaneously or in response to my inquiries (but not by bragging and talking incessantly and irrelevantly).

_____12. The therapist encourages a feeling that I am as good as he/she is.

_____13. The therapist acts as if he/she is my consultant, rather than the manager of my life.

_____14. The therapist encourages differences of opinion rather than telling me that I am resisting if I disagree with him/her.

_____15. The therapist is interested in seeing people who share my life (or is at least willing to do so). This would include family, friends, lovers, work associates, or any other significant people in my envorinment.

_____16. The things that the therapist says make sense to me.

_____17. In general, my contacts with the therapist lead to my feeling more hopeful and having higher self-esteem.

_____TOTAL

Interpreting your score. You would probably not feel comfortable working with a therapist who rated below 50 points. Certainly, you should not even consider working with someone whose score fell below 40 points. Don't hesitate to see several therapists betore choosing one.

Also, decisions are not irrevocable. Don't think you have to stay with a particular therapist simply because you have started or have been with the same person for months or even years. It is your time, money, and well-being that are at stake. If you have tried several therapists with different styles and personalities and none seems satisfactory, perhaps it is better to work with one who has the highest score rather than using an absolute figure.

Even after visiting a specific therapist for several sessions, you can still change therapists if you are not making progress or if the therapist is not going in the direction you desire. Remember, the therapist always works for you! You are the boss and must call the shots. If you want help with your binge-purge problem, but the therapist insists that you must work on your relationship with your mother, beat a hasty retreat and find someone else. The days are long gone when the therapist must be treated as the "Great White Doctor." Second and third options are acceptable with medical problems, so why not with psychological problems? To help you better understand your relationship with your therapist, consider the following list of Client Rights suggested by the California State Psychological Association.

1. You have the right to decide not to receive psychotherapy from me; if you wish, I shall provide you with the names of other qualified psychotherapists.

2. You have the right to prevent the use of certain procedures used during therapy; if you wish, I shall explain any unusual procedures.

3. You have the right to prevent the use of certain therapeutic techniques; I shall inform you of my intention to use any usual procedures and shall describe any risks involved.

4. You have the right to prevent electronic recording of any part of the therapy sessions; permission to record must be granted by you in writing on a form that explains what is to be done and for what period of time. I shall explain my intended use of the recordings and provide a written statement to the effect that they will not be used for any other purpose; you have the right to withdraw your permission to record at any time.

5. You have the right to review your records in the files at any time.

6. If you request it, any part of your record in the files can be released to any person or agencies you designate. I shall tell you, at the time, whether or not I think making the record public will be harmful to you.

7. One of your most important rights involves confidentiality: within certain limits, information revealed by you during therapy will be kept strictly confidential and will not be revealed to any other person or agency without your written permission. One exception to this rule would be the failure on your part to pay the clinical fee. This default on your part may result in the release of your name and other relevant information to a private collection agency.

8. You should also know that there are certain situations in which, as a psychotherapist, I am required by law to reveal information obtained during therapy to other persons or agencies—*without your permission.* Also, I am not required to inform you of my actions in this regard. These situations are as follows:

a. If you threaten grave bodily harm or death to another person, I am required by law to inform the intended victim and appropriate law enforcement agencies;

b. if a court of law issues a legitimate subpoena, I am required by law to provide the information specifically described in the subpoena;

c. if you are in therapy or being tested by order of a court of law, the results of the treatment or tests ordered must be revealed to the court.

Bibliography

Arenson, G. *How to Stop Playing the Weighting Game*. Los Angeles: Transformation Publications, 1978.

Bach, G. *The Inner Enemy*. New York: Morrow, 1983.

Backus, W., and Chapian, M. *Telling Yourself the Truth*. Minneapolis: Bethany House Publishers, 1981.

Bailey, C. *Fit or Fat?* Boston: Houghton Mifflin, 1978.

Bruch, H. *The Golden Cage*. New York: Vintage Books, 1979.

Burka, J. B., and Lenora, Y. M. *Procrastination*. Menlo Park, CA: Addison-Wesley, 1983.

Burns, D. *Feeling Good: The New Mood Therapy*. New York: Morrow, 1980.

Burns, D. *Intimate Connections*. New York: Morrow, 1985.

Caplan, G., and Killilea, M., eds. *Support Systems and Mutual Help*. New York: Gruen & Stratton, 1976.

Davis, M.; Eshelman, E. R.; and McKay, M. *The Relaxation & Stress Reduction Workbook*. Oakland, CA: New Harbinger Publications, Inc., 1982.

Dowling, C. *The Cinderella Complex*. New York: Pocket Books, 1981.

Dyer, W. *Your Erroneous Zones*. New York: Funk & Wagnalls, 1976.

Ellis, A., and Harper, R. A. *A New Guide to Rational Living*. New York: Prentice-Hall, 1975.

Evans, G. *The Family Circle Guide to Self-Help*. New York: Ballantine, 1979.

Fensterheim, H., and Baer, J. *Don't Say Yes When You Want to Say No*. New York: Dell, 1975.

Garfinkel, P. E., and Garner, D. M. *Anorexia Nervosa: A Multidimensional Perspective*. New York: Brunner Mazel, 1982.

Hodgson, R., and Miller, P. *Self-Watching*. London: Multimedia Publications, 1982.

Houston, J. P. *The Pursuit of Happiness*. Palo Alto, CA: Scott, Foresman, 1981.

Kroger, W. S., and Fezler, W. D. *Hypnosis and Behavior Modification: Imagery Conditioning*. Philadelphia: Lippincott, 1976.

Lakein, A. *How to Get Control of Your Time and Your Life*. New York: Signet, 1973.

Lazarus, A. *I Can If I Want to*. New York: Warner, 1977.

Martin, R. A., and Poland, E. Y. *Learning to Change*. New York: McGraw Hill, 1980.

McKay, M.; Davis, M.; and Fanning, P. *Messages: The Communication Book*. Oakland, CA: New Harbinger Publications, 1983.

McMullin, R., and Casey, B. *Talk Sense to Yourself*. Lakewood, CO: Counseling Research Institute, 1975.

Miller, P. M. *Personal Habit Control*. New York: Simon and Schuster, 1978.

Neuman, P. A., and Halvorson, P. A. *Anorexia Nervosa and Bulimia*. New York: Von Nostrand, 1983.

Orbach, S. *Fat is a Feminist Issue*. New York: Berkeley Publishing Company, 1978.

Polivy, J., and Herman, C. P. *Breaking the Diet Habit: The Natural Weight Alternative*. New York: Basic Books, 1983.

Rachman, S. J., and Hodgson, R. *Obsessions and Compulsions*. Englewood-Cliffs, NJ: Prentice-Hall, 1980.

Robinson, D., and Henry, S. *Self-Help and Health: Mutual Aid for Modern Problems*. London: Croom Helm, 1977.

Russianoff, P. *Why Do I Think I am Nothing Without a Man?* New York: Bantam Books, 1982.

Seabury, D. *The Art of Selfishness*. New York: Pocket Books, 1964.

Sehnert, K. W. *Stress/Unstress*. Minneapolis: Augsburg, 1981.

Slochower, J. A. *Excessive Eating: The Role of Emotions and Environment*. New York: Human Sciences Press, 1983.

Travis, J. W. *Wellness Workbook*. Mill Valley, CA: Wellness Associates, 1977.

Watson, D. L., and Tharp, R. G. *Self-Directed Behavior*. Monterey, CA: Brooks/Cole, 1981.

Wilson, R. "Analyzing the daily risks of life," *Technical Review*, Feb. 1979.

Zimbardo, P. E. *Shyness*. Menlo Park, CA: Addison-Wesley, 1978.

Other New Harbinger Self-Help Titles

Last Touch: Preparing for a Parents Death, $11.95
Consuming Passions: Help for Compulsive Shoppers, $11.95
Self-Esteem, Second Edition, $12.95
Depression & Anxiety Mangement: An audio tape for managing emotional problems, $11.95
I Can't Get Over It, A Handbook for Trauma Survivors, $12.95
Concerned Intervention, When Your Loved One Won't Quit Alcohol or Drugs, $11.95
Redefining Mr. Right, $11.95
Dying of Embarrassment: Help for Social Anxiety and Social Phobia, $11.95
The Depression Workbook: Living With Depression and Manic Depression, $13.95
Risk-Taking for Personal Growth: A Step-by-Step Workbook, $11.95
The Marriage Bed: Renewing Love, Friendship, Trust, and Romance, $11.95
Focal Group Psychotherapy: For Mental Health Professionals, $44.95
Hot Water Therapy: Save Your Back, Neck & Shoulders in 10 Minutes a Day $11.95
Older & Wiser: A Workbook for Coping With Aging, $12.95
Prisoners of Belief: Exposing & Changing Beliefs that Control Your Life, $10.95
Be Sick Well: A Healthy Approach to Chronic Illness, $11.95
Men & Grief: A Guide for Men Surviving the Death of a Loved One., $11.95
When the Bough Breaks: A Guide for Parents of Sexually Abused Childern, $11.95
Love Addiction: A Guide to Emotional Independence, $11.95
When Once Is Not Enough: Help for Obsessive Compulsives, $11.95
The New Three Minute Meditator, $9.95
Getting to Sleep, $10.95
The Relaxation & Stress Reduction Workbook, 3rd Edition, $13.95
Leader's Guide to the Relaxation & Stress Reduction Workbook, $19.95
Beyond Grief: A Guide for Recovering from the Death of a Loved One, $10.95
Thoughts & Feelings: The Art of Cognitive Stress Intervention, $13.95
Messages: The Communication Skills Book, $12.95
The Divorce Book, $11.95
Hypnosis for Change: A Manual of Proven Techniques, 2nd Edition, $12.95
The Deadly Diet: Recovering from Anorexia & Bulimia, $11.95
Chronic Pain Control Workbook, $13.95
Rekindling Desire: Bringing Your Sexual Relationship Back to Life, $12.95
Life Without Fear: Anxiety and Its Cure, $10.95
Visualization for Change, $12.95
Guideposts to Meaning: Discovering What Really Matters, $11.95
Videotape: Clinical Hypnosis for Stress & Anxiety Reduction, $24.95
Starting Out Right: Essential Parenting Skills for Your Child's First Seven Years, $12.95
Big Kids: A Parent's Guide to Weight Control for Children, $11.95
My Parent's Keeper: Adult Children of the Emotionally Disturbed, $11.95
When Anger Hurts, $12.95
Free of the Shadows: Recovering from Sexual Violence, $12.95
Resolving Conflict With Others and Within Yourself, $12.95
Lifetime Weight Control, $11.95
The Anxiety & Phobia Workbook, $13.95
Love and Renewal: A Couple's Guide to Commitment, $12.95
The Habit Control Workbook, $12.95

Call **toll free, 1-800-748-6273**, to order books. Have your Visa or Mastercard number ready. Or send a check for the titles you want to New Harbinger Publications, 5674 Shattuck Avenue, Oakland, CA 94609. Include $2.00 for the first book and 50¢ for each additional book, to cover shipping and handling. (California residents please include appropriate sales tax.) Allow four to six weeks for delivery.

Prices subject to change without notice.